LETTERS TO MY
BROWN MOTHER

LETTERS TO MY BROWN MOTHER

STORIES OF MENTAL HEALTH

MUZNA ABBAS

NEW DEGREE PRESS

COPYRIGHT © 2021 MUZNA ABBAS

LETTERS TO MY BROWN MOTHER
Stories of Mental Health

ISBN   978-1-63730-623-9   *Hardcover*

978-1-63730-353-5   *Paperback*

978-1-63730-354-2   *Kindle Ebook*

978-1-63730-355-9   *Ebook*

to Mama and Papa

Table of Contents

THE STIGMA

PART 1.   **SETTING THE SCENE**
ABCD | AMERICAN-BORN CONFUSED DESI
THE INVISIBLE CRISIS

PART 2.   **THE STORIES WE NEVER TOLD**
POSTER CHILD
LOG KYA KAHENGE? | WHAT WILL PEOPLE SAY?
SANDWICH GENERATION
FAMILY HEIRLOOMS
MARDANGI | MANHOOD
AMMI KI GURIYA | MY MOTHER'S DOLL
PRIDE

PART 3.   **MOVING FORWARD**
SELF-CARE
THERAPY
BOUNDARIES
DIFFICULT CONVERSATIONS
THE CHARGE AHEAD

you are lonely

but you are not alone

there is a difference

-RUPI KAUR

The Stigma

Dear Reader,

The first time I spoke the words out loud, I was in tears and my voice was barely audible. I had been crying alone for an hour, walking aimlessly around campus. Finally, my roommates found me sitting on a poorly lit bench overlooking the canyon. I had no excuse to give them for my crying. "School is stressing me out," had been used too many times.

I talked in circles and didn't give a straight answer. I couldn't look them in the eye, so instead I continued picking the red paint of the wooden bench. I heard their consoling voices, but I wasn't paying much attention to their actual words. I wanted to tell them; I had to. My mouth opened a few times in between a "You're going to get through this" and a "You're not alone" to speak, but words failed to come out. Suddenly, as if it were someone else in my body, I interrupted one of my roommates—

"The doctor gave me pills for depression." I waited to see disapproving looks of disgust or pity on their faces. Instead, they hugged me tightly. I felt safe and protected, at ease. I hadn't felt such emotions in a long time.

Before this, I had projected my own shame and embarrassment over my diagnosis of depression and internalized the stigma around antidepressant medication. I felt the same disdain for myself that I had always seen from others about the "crazy people who were on pills." *I guess that's me now.*

But when I opened myself up to my friends, I was pleasantly surprised at their reactions. I felt better than I anticipated, which gave me the hope and courage to tell my mother about my new reality. I decided to do it that night, unsure when I'd ever have the courage to talk about this again.

I walked back to my dorm room with my roommates and sat on my bottom-bunk bed in my cramped freshman triple. I took a deep breath and hit the button. As soon as I heard the first ring my hands began to shake. *Am I really doing this? I should just hang up.*

"Hello!" My heart sank when I heard her voice. *I can't to do this. Abort mission.* She asked about my day and I reflexively went through the motions of small talk about school and friends and everything in between. *Thankfully she can't see how puffy my eyes are.*

The orange prescription bottle on my nightstand stared intently at me, as if trying to tell me: "Do it already!" *Fine, I'll do it.*

"I went to the doctor a few weeks ago. She diagnosed me with severe depression, which I guess is a mental disorder. She said that's why I've been feeling so down and not myself lately. I had been missing a lot of classes because I didn't feel like going. All I wanted to do was sleep. I didn't know what to do. The doctor said the depression is probably the reason for that. She gave me some medication, antidepressant pills, that are supposed to make me feel better. I've been taking them for a few weeks now." I said it all in one breath. I didn't want any pauses in between to invite questions.

She took a second to answer. "Depression? What are you sad about? You're going to a great college; you're getting good grades. Are you upset with someone? Did you have a fight with someone? What could you be sad about? You know this is probably happening because you've stopped praying since you started college. You need to pray more. That will fix your sadness." My mom diagnosed me in less time than my doctor had.

I didn't really know how to react to her response, and I had a feeling whatever else she would say wasn't going to make me feel better. This conversation didn't go like it had with my roommates.

"I don't really know. I've already tried praying." I sighed. "It's getting late, I have an eight a.m. class tomorrow. I should go to bed."

"Oh, okay." She sighed in response. "Goodnight, then."

I picked up a book to distract my mind with its printed words. I turned pages fast, though not comprehending anything Stephen Chbosky had to say about wallflowers.

I didn't get the reaction I hoped for when discussing my mental health with my Pakistani family. Instead, I was met with the same embarrassment, denial, and pity I had been projecting onto myself. Mental wellbeing was never something we discussed in my house growing up. It wasn't until I was sitting in the doctor's office that I heard about depression as a mental health issue. That is exactly what I hope to change with this book.

Countless times throughout this journey, I was reminded of the necessity and urgency for someone to tell the stories of South Asian-Americans and their mental health. These stories detail our unique upbringing as third-culture kids or, as some liked to say, ABCDs (American-Born Confused Desi). While we've been gaining representation in the media, there's a long way to go to reach *authentic* representation. That's why this book is necessary—to represent us in *all* the ways we come, including the good, the bad, and even the ugly. At times this task felt awfully daunting, but I fought through the fear and hesitation because I knew who was on the other side: you.

I wrote this book for you. I wrote this book for those of you who suffered mental health issues in silence, for those who helplessly watched someone you care about suffer. This book is for those of you who did not know how to seek help, where to seek help, or if that help was even there. I wrote this book for those who have lost loved ones to mental health struggles. I wrote for those of you who want to help: yourself, your friends, your parents, and your children. I wrote this book for you. But I also wrote this book for me and my eighteen-year-old self. I wrote this book as an advocate, a survivor, a child of immigrants, and, someday, a parent.

The stories and experiences detailed within these pages are from real South Asian-Americans. While their names may be changed and some details exaggerated, the emotions are true, authentic, and raw. I hope you will be as moved as I was when I listened to them recount their journeys. To those of you who shared, I thank you from the bottom my heart for your vulnerability and openness. I thank you for trusting me with pieces of your lived experience and for letting me share them with the world. I was left inspired by your strength and courage to speak your truths and face your fears.

As you read this book, I hope you, too, can see why this conversation is needed, and needed *now*. This book is only the start of that conversation: a fraction of the experiences and realities of South Asian-Americans. These are their stories and my interpretations. There are still unspoken truths out there, unheard voices. I hope this book will allow them a safe community and platform to make their voices heard. Lastly, I hope we can normalize dealing with mental health struggles and taking care of them—no matter who you are or where you come from.

Enjoy,
Muzna

Don't be a baby • You're just making it up •
Stop being lazy • You're not working hard
enough • You need to pray more • Stop trying to get attention • *Dramay-baaz* • *Jhoo-
tih* • *Jhootah* • You're crazy • *Pagal* • Don't
tell anybody • Someone must have cast the
evil eye on you • *Nazar lag gaye hai* • What
will people say? • *Log kya kahenge?*

Any mention of struggles with mental health in a South
Asian[1] household will yield one of the above responses, or
something similar. When young people try to discuss mental
health with their parents or family, their concerns are often
dismissed. Whether out of denial, shame, or lack of understanding, mental health is taboo and seldom discussed in
South Asian communities.

According to the CDC, in 2019, suicide was the leading
cause of death for Asian-Americans between ten and twenty-four years old (CDC, 2020). Other research shows Asian
Americans are less likely to use mental health services than
Caucasians, even though the likelihood of experiencing psychological distress is comparable (US DHHS, 2001). In a 2010

---

1   I identify South Asians as those who ethnically originate from the following countries: Afghanistan, Bangladesh, Bhutan, India, Nepal, Pakistan,
Sri Lanka, and the Maldives.

study of college students, Loya, Reddy, and Hinshaw found South Asians, specifically, demonstrated a greater reluctance than their Caucasian peers toward using mental health-related counseling services. They also found South Asians to have higher levels of personal stigma toward mental illness, like I used to have. If the rates of experiencing depression or social anxiety is comparable to other racial groups, why are Asian-Americans, South Asians in particular, seeking and utilizing mental health services at far lower rates?

Stigma.

The negative stigma surrounding mental health issues is rooted deep into the sociocultural fabric of South Asian culture, especially within immigrant communities. When mental health is brought up, the only options are to ignore it, deem it false, or—in the rare and extreme cases where it is addressed—keep it secret. But just because these issues are ignored, not believed, or hidden doesn't mean they cease to exist. They exist and they cause real harm.

When mental health issues are unaddressed or unaccepted, individuals seek unhealthy coping mechanisms that end up causing more harm. Unexamined mental distress can cause a rapid decline in mental health, as well as a higher likelihood of dangerous and abusive behaviors. Leaving these issues untreated can lead to a longer, more uncertain, and costlier road to recovery. Many turn to drugs and alcohol, but these coping mechanisms can quickly turn into substance abuse. Others turn to self-harming behaviors such as intentional cutting, burning, or scratching. All of these unhealthy coping mechanisms further deteriorate poor mental health: cue a destructive downward spiral.

The societal discomfort surrounding mental health not only prevents people from seeking help, but also prevents them from understanding their own mental health concerns are legitimate. The Substance Abuse and Mental Health Services Administration notes Asian-Americans (the category most South Asians identify as) are the least likely ethnic group to reach out for help when it comes to their mental health.

When my doctor first diagnosed me with depression, I didn't ask many questions or try to understand what it all meant out of shame and fear. I didn't really want to know exactly what was happening to me—the more I knew, the more concrete it would become. For the longest time, I kept myself from understanding my diagnosis and how to manage it. My own preconceived views of depression, derived from the community I grew up in, restrained me from discussing my situation with others or seeking support. I didn't want to be that girl seeing a "shrink," or known as someone who had to take pills to survive. I especially did not want to be that depressed girl who killed herself.

Negative and rigid views of depression made the first couple months after diagnosis grueling. I beat myself up over "what I had become," only making matters worse. I was in denial and alone because talking about it with anyone wasn't an option. When I did talk about it, the responses I received from my family weren't the ones I needed to hear.

"This is probably happening because you've stopped praying since you started college. You need to pray more. That will fix your sadness," my mom had said.

Like for many others who have heard something similar, a statement that was probably meant to be reassuring and helpful didn't feel as such. I remember thinking: *God is punishing me. This is my fault and I have to live with the consequences.*

Depression and anxiety were foreign concepts to my parents, something they barely believed to be real. After all, how could their high-achieving, successful daughter be sad? What could she be sad about? After that discussion with my mom, I didn't bring up my mental health or anything else that was bothering me to my family again. What was the point? I would only be blamed for the problems I had. I already felt hopeless and despondent; why discuss it and make myself feel even worse? Case closed.

As a family-driven culture, we would be remiss for not taking care of our family members. Why, then, do we fail to take care of our family when they suffer from mental health issues? Why does family not come first when anxiety, depression, and other mental illnesses are in the room? Addressing mental health challenges is crucial, and it starts with understanding what it is and where it comes from. With this book, I hope to do just that.

As I write this during a pandemic, mental health is more important than ever—more fragile than ever. Through this book, I hope to share the mental health stories of the South Asian diaspora, especially with our parents. It's necessary to not only tell these stories, but also to provide a roadmap for the future. I share others' experiences as well as my own to help people, like my younger self, understand they're not alone. They can get help and deserve to feel better.

This book is for eighteen-year-old me and those like her who struggled to come to terms with their mental health issues. I hope to make the conversation immigrant children have with their parents about mental health easier for everyone involved. Dismantling stigma will enable us to openly have crucial conversations about mental health and wellness so we're able to get the help we need. I'm confident that by starting this societal conversation on mental health in the South Asian diaspora, we can do better for our future generations.

WHAT COMES NEXT

In order to remove this stigma and reluctance to acknowledge and take care of our mental health, we must first understand what it looks like. The only way to truly comprehend the influence and weight of this burden is by learning from others' experiences. I hope to rely on the power of storytelling to allow an intimate and personal glimpse into the struggles fellow South Asians have experienced with their mental health. It's only by seeing these struggles from the inside can we begin to recognize how they present on the outside.

This book is divided into three parts. In Part One, I start by setting the scene to introduce who we are, as South Asians, and the invisible crisis we're facing. A brief history of South Asian immigration and culture, as well as an overview of mental health conditions, will help contextualize our collective experiences.

You will find a series of letters, inspired by real South Asian-American's stories, in Part Two. Some letters are written to our mothers, some to our fathers, and some to ourselves. You'll hear from young adults, parents, children, elders, professionals, and even myself. All these unique, individual stories will help us understand the collective experience of South Asian immigrants and their mental health. Each chapter will cover a cultural theme or phenomena that either negatively affects mental health in our communities or further deepens the stigma toward it. Among these are: generational trauma, guilt and shame, toxic masculinity, misogynistic gender roles, and more.

Part Three discusses how we can protect our mental health and move forward. I present several strategies recommended and studied by medical professionals, some of which I have used. This last part of the book also details how we can have the difficult conversation on mental health with our loved ones. Having these conversations isn't only another mechanism to take care of our mental health, but it's also an opportunity for us to break the stigma within our society.

By the end, I hope you're left with three things: 1) a deeper understanding of the mental health experiences of fellow South Asians, 2) better tactics to take care of your mental health, and 3) a model—and hopefully the will—for having difficult conversations about mental health.

In this book, I will often use the word *Desi* (*they-see*) to collectively describe South Asians. This word personally holds a lot of significance, as it evokes a sense of community and belongingness that "Asian" or "South Asian" simply do not. Desi comes from the Sanskrit word *desh,* meaning country, and refers to someone or something native to a country. The term Desi reminds me of how our identity and roots have traveled from our homelands, our *desh,* around the world with us. It is a term we should blazon with pride regardless of the combination of colors our flag happens to be painted with.

Some have argued Desi is a reductive term that assumes we are "indiscriminately homogenous, or worse, that we understand each other's cultures completely" (Guha, 2013). But I believe the term Desi is *our* word to define—we get to decide what it means. Desi can be our version of reclaiming our race like the Black Lives Matter Movement has reclaimed Black as a term to be celebrated and an identity to be proud of (Lamonier, 2019). The Black experience is not homogenous for every Black person; the Desi experience doesn't have to be either. Shared identity evokes a shared experience, a common bond that can be small or large.

Anyone who identifies with the South Asian ethnic heritage unequivocally shares a small or large bond with others who also identify as such. *Desi* connects us to something bigger than ourselves and it softens the (rigid) lines carved into a subcontinent that was (mostly) at peace with and reveled in its diversity. By claiming ourselves as Desis and bringing our diverse cultures to the table, we can reclaim this term to represent our rich, complex, and expansive South Asian experience.

For me, a native Urdu speaker, language played a significant part in shaping my identity. It connects me with my culture, and I want you to feel that connection with me. I've included a glossary of terms at the end that clarifies some of the Hindi/Urdu/Bangla words or phrases I use, and other terminology scattered throughout the book. The definitions in the glossary are my interpretations of the language I grew up around. Your interpretations might be different, and you might not agree with mine, but that's the beauty of language.

Finally, I want to say: this book is not meant to demonize our cultures. This is my culture and I *love* it—I take pride in it. Nevertheless, much of what I say remains critical of our culture. This critique is important and necessary because *we can do better!* We *must* do better. If we don't, we will keep driving our own people away from this beautiful culture. There are already so many of us who feel suffocated by the rigidity of our culture and find it necessary to shun their "Desi" side. If that continues to happen, the South Asian heritage that made us who we are will slowly become extinct. If our culture keeps harming and hurting the mental health of future generations, more and more people will decide to erase their South Asian identities. And that would be the real shame.

PART ONE:

SETTING THE SCENE

"I am from there. I am from here. I am not there and I am not here. I have two names, which meet and part, and I have two languages. I forget which of them I dream in."

-MAHMOUD DARWISH

ABCD | American-Born Confused Desi

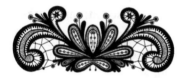

WHO WE ARE:

"India clings to me, as she does to all her
children, in innumerable ways."

-JAWAHARLAL NEHRU (INDIA'S FIRST PRIME MINISTER)

Nehru's above sentiment is actually applicable to all South
Asian diasporic communities. Whether they immigrated for
family or a career, South Asians have maintained a desire to
preserve their ethnic and cultural identity wherever they go.
While the various practiced religions bring nuance to some of
these cultural values, the broader South Asian culture shares

many roots in that it is a collectivist culture: one that places the family or tribal unit at its core. Most Asian and African cultures tend to be more collectivist while Western (European) cultures are more individualistic. In contrast to individualism where personal freedom and characteristics are emphasized, collectivism values personal *inter*dependence. Such a culture "encourages conformity and discourages individuals from dissenting and standing out," focusing on the embeddedness of individuals within their family (Gorodnichenko and Roland, 2012). In collective cultures, the family unit's needs supersede the desires of an individual.

As such, the culture is also extremely prescriptive. There is a cultural, religious, or societal reason or solution for every situation. The fundamentals of many of these cultural "commandments" include:

- Self-respect, dignity, and self-control: "From early childhood, the importance of these three variables is emphasized. Each person is empowered to achieve self-respect, dignity, and self-control. The person is seen as an individual [within] a familial context. Individuality of a person is encouraged [only] within the boundaries and limits of the family" (Ibrahim et al, 1997). In practice this enforces a restraint on expression of one's personality, especially in public. *Sharam*, modesty, and a general temperateness is expected.
- Respect for the family above all else: Parents and all elders are to be respected, revered, and obeyed. The family unit is sacred; family (even extended family) always comes first. To keep this extended family unit intact, many families choose to live in *joint-family systems*. While this

is difficult to pull off financially in the US, immigrant families tend to have multigenerational households with grandparents, parents, children, and even grandchildren living together.

- Respect for age: Elders are respected for their wisdom and knowledge; they simply know better. Families turn to their elders for advice, which they are then expected to follow.
- Respect for community: The cultural community is seen as an extension of the family for most immigrants. As such, one has responsibilities to their community as well. This requires the maintenance of respect, self-control, and honor within the community, often at any cost.
- Hierarchy: The South Asian culture highly regards hierarchy in social relationships. Your placement within the hierarchy is determined not only by age, but also by gender, family relationships, education, and social class. The emphasis placed on hierarchies reinforces the principle that individualism is secondary to the importance of the group. Gender often precedes most other categories, even age, within the hierarchical structure.

Because of the heavy value placed on the family unit and community, outward appearances and perceptions are extremely important and must always be well-maintained. A public restraint on emotions, feelings, and thoughts is expected to portray a pristine image of harmony (whether it exists or not). Unpleasant topics or disagreements are never to be had in public or in front of other members of the community. This obsession over reputation within the community tends to cause friction between parents and children.

Patriarchy is another key pillar of Desi culture. Per its most basic definition, patriarchy refers to a social system where men are the head of the family, holding the power in political, moral, and social realms (Das and Kemp, 1997). While the oppression of women is not an explicit trait of a patriarchal system, it is a direct consequence of it. In a male-dominated society, there are strict gender norms restricting everyone, males and females, into their predefined roles in society. There is also no space for a spectrum of gender to exist within this rigid dichotomy.

Traditionally, a woman's role is restricted to the domestic sphere: she must know how to take care of and raise a family. Expectations for women are that they stay home and follow the lead of the household's men. Women and girls are required to be feminine and prepare for marriage. Men, on the other hand, are expected to be strong heads of house, with little room for emotions. They are the breadwinners, their masculinity tied to their financial success. While some of these norms may not be as strictly practiced in all immigrant communities, their shadows linger and can be seen through other cultural practices and norms.

Deeply connected to gender roles and expectations, religion is another cornerstone of South Asian culture. It's one that plays a major role in everyone's lives, whether they choose to practice religion or not. Whether Sikh, Hindu, Muslim, Buddhist, or Christian, South Asians define their identity by their religion. It's so foundational to how we see ourselves that the extent of our piety is directly tied to our worth and acceptance in society, particularly for women. You're a good daughter if you're a devout [insert religion here]. Gender and religion go hand in hand, with the bulk of religious duties falling on women.

Much of the culture is derived from the religions that are practiced. So, the lines between religion and culture are blurred. Cultural practices are given religious justifications and religious practices are blended with cultural ones. This entanglement of religion and culture, while promoting strong faith, leaves little room for personal interpretation or choice. Denouncing culture means you are inevitably denouncing religion and vice versa. And denouncing religion is akin to denouncing your identity and your worth.

As mentioned earlier, collectivist cultures require a high degree of social *inter*dependence. Individuality isn't celebrated, nor is it generally accepted. In the South Asian culture, "people are born into groups—families, clans, subcastes, castes, and religious communities—and live with a constant sense of being part of and inseparable from these groups" (Heitzman and Woorden, 1996). In such a society, the concept of privacy is incomprehensible. In fact, privacy is often considered a privilege, something only the wealthy can have. Neither modern Hindi nor Urdu languages have a word to represent the exact concept of privacy. There are words that describe isolation, secrecy, or loneliness, but nothing that describes the right to be left alone (Kumar, 2017). When there aren't exact words to describe a concept, it points to a conceptual ambiguity: that particular concept doesn't exist.

Consequently, privacy is a rare phenomenon in Desi culture. Your business is your family's business and your family's business is your business. Asking for or expecting privacy isn't easy to do, especially between parents and children. With this lack of privacy comes a lack of personal boundaries as well. The interdependent family structure means individuality isn't respected. You aren't seen as the individual you are but based on your role in the family dynamic. You're the "daughter," the "son," or the "mother." The stripping away of your identity and lack of boundaries in the family translate to *enmeshment*. When personal boundaries are blurred, everyone's feelings, identities, and needs bleed into each other. Independence is stifled and the family's needs are prioritized over those of the individual.

HOW WE GOT HERE:

Historically, South Asians have been immigrating to North America since the early twentieth century. These migrants settled in the US as: 1) laborers for the Western Pacific Railroad, 2) merchants and traders, and 3) university students. During World War One, Indian migrants enlisted and served in the US Army. Indians, who could pass for and identify as "white," were even able to become naturalized US citizens. But the anti-immigrant sentiment that grew in the aftermath of the war made that path to citizenship difficult for many, especially those who were assumed to be from "The East." In the 1923 case of *US v. Bhagat Singh Thind*, the Supreme Court unanimously voted to cancel Thind's naturalization, claiming he was not "Caucasian in the common understanding" so he didn't qualify as a "free white person" outlined in the Naturalization Act of 1906. It was decided "Hindus [were] Too Brunette To Vote": the verdict deemed South Asians ineligible for naturalization and revoked the citizenships of many Indian-Americans, forcing them to go back to India (*The Literary Digest*, 1923).

Even though the population of South Asians in the US was small during this time, heavy xenophobia lead to anti-Indian riots and the growing fear of a "Hindoo Invasion" post-World War One (Maira, 2002). In response to this anti-Asiatic sentiment, an immigration restriction law was also passed in 1917 and designated India as part of the "Asiatic barred zone," from which immigration to the US was prohibited. Despite the inability to obtain citizenship, some of the Indian immigrants suffered through the racism and discrimination and chose to stay, but many fled back home and others were forcefully deported from the US.

On the other side of the world, in the 1930s, Gandhi's nonviolent independence campaigns against Britain's two-hundred-year-long oppressive rule in India were taking shape. The movement Gandhi ignited and the rising tensions between Hindus and Muslims ultimately led to the independence from British rule in 1947. At that time, British India was divided into majority Hindu India and majority Muslim Pakistan: borders were drawn up overnight. An estimated twelve to eighteen million people migrated between the two newly created nations as Muslims moved east from India to Pakistan and Hindus and Sikhs moved westward from Pakistan to India. This mass migration, the largest in human history, was riddled with bloodshed and violence. Keys in hand, many families left their homes locked up and had hoped to return, but they never survived the trek to the other side. As the wounds of the 1947 partition began to scab over, many began to look outward for better opportunities abroad.

The Immigration and Nationality Act of 1965 propelled South Asian immigration to the US as it replaced the old immigration system (established in 1924) that was based on racial and national quotas. This new system gave preference to immigrants who: already had family in the US (for family reunification), were fleeing persecution (to claim refugee status), or worked in specific, highly-demanded professions (brought work-related skills).

The Cold War encouraged the immigration of professionals with skills in technology and medicine, leading to a boom of high-skilled South Asian immigrants. Thus, post-1965 South Asian immigrants were educated, with advanced degrees in medicine, law, and other STEM fields. The family reunification immigration classification also drove many immigrants to the US and helped create the large pockets of South Asian communities that exist today in New York City, the San Francisco Bay Area, Chicago, Houston, and Dallas. The past two decades have seen larger spikes of South Asian immigration due to the increased cap of the H-1B visa limit to one hundred ninety-five thousand from 2001 to 2003.[2] The influx of highly educated South Asians, and Asian immigrants in general, with high median incomes and fluency in English forged the "model minority" image, which will be discussed later in the book.

The Pew Research Center divides immigrant families into three categories:

---

2   This cap reverted back to the original sixty-five thousand in 2004.

- **First generation**: Foreign-born immigrants who now live in the United States and/or are naturalized US citizens.
- **Second generation**: US-born children of at least one foreign-born, immigrant parent.
- **Third and higher generation:** Children of US-born parents.

While these delineations make sense from a historical and research perspective, they fail to encapsulate the unique experiences of the identified second generation, those who are US-born but have foreign-born parents. The term "second generation" implies the first generation also had the opportunity to grow up in the United States. For many of us, that is not the case. In most instances, the second generation is the first of the family that is raised in America and truly experiences both cultures (American and their ethnic culture) while growing up. This experience is vastly different from children whose parents were also raised (or partially raised) in the US.

The second generation is typically the first one to navigate the K–12 educational system and college in America, which can be difficult coming from a household that didn't always understand the system. For example, while buying a house, my parents weren't aware of the importance of school districts when picking a location—that knowledge comes from understanding a system from within. The Pew-delineated second generation should actually be considered the first generation since we are the first ones to come of age and form our identities in the context of two cultures.

For this book, I will use the following categories to define the generations:

- **Immigrant generation**: This applies to my parents who were born and raised in Pakistan and immigrated to the US as adults.
- **First generation**: This refers my sisters and I who were born in the US to immigrant parents. This also applies to my peers who may not have been born here, but were raised and grew up here.
- **Second and higher generations**: This will apply to mine and my sisters' future children who will have at least one parent who was born or raised in the US to immigrant parents.

The Invisible Crisis

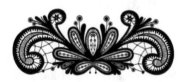

WHAT WE'RE DEALING WITH

Millions of people around the globe deal with mental health issues every year. In 2019, one in five adults (roughly 51.5 million) in the US experienced mental distress (NAMI, 2021). There are many different mental disorders that range in their severity and treatment strategies. The most common among these are depression, anxiety, eating disorders, and post-traumatic stress disorders. Other disorders include: schizophrenia, bipolar disorder, borderline personality disorder, and obsessive-compulsive disorder.

All mental health conditions affect an individual's mood, behavior, feelings, and thinking, which causes overall distress and difficulty in functioning. Changes in mental health affect your daily activities such as maintaining relationships, productivity (school, work, caregiving), and taking care of yourself.

The onset of a mental health condition is not the result of one event, but a combination of several things: inherited traits, environmental factors, lifestyle, and brain chemistry.

Certain genes are correlated with higher risk of developing mental illness, especially when blood relatives also have similar conditions. The environment you grow up in has a tremendous effect on the development of mental health issues. Environmental risk factors include abuse and neglect during childhood, traumatic experiences, and exposure to toxins, alcohol, and drugs in the womb or during childhood. Lifestyle changes and stressors such as a loss of a loved one, a stressful job, or an unstable household can also trigger mental health conditions.

Harvard psychologist Richard McNally confirms mental illnesses are partly rooted in the brain's anatomy (Weir, 2012). The chemicals, called neurotransmitters, that carry signals to your brain and body travel on neural networks and communicate with nerve receptors. If these neurotransmitters are in short supply or can't reach the correct nerve receptor, the key chemicals associated with happiness, motivation, and responding to stress (fight-or-flight responses) don't reach the brain when and where they should. This chemical imbalance prevents the brain from communicating effectively with the body, inhibiting an appropriate response to the stimulus around us. Other complications can also arise because of issues with nerve cell connections, nerve cell growth, and the overall functioning of nerve circuits, as they're all part of the brain circuit. These "software bugs" in our brains can cause several types of mental conditions that include: mood disorders, anxiety disorders, eating disorders, and post-traumatic stress disorder, among others.

When we first think of mental health, our immediate thought goes toward depression. Mood disorders, such as depression, affect our motivation and emotional connections. For example, people struggling with mood disorders can either appear overly sad, show a lack of emotion, and be inappropriately happy or energetic at the wrong time. The disorder is an inability to regulate these moods. Imagine someone happy at a funeral (manic episode/bipolar disorder) or someone so sad or unmotivated they can't find the energy to get out of bed in the morning.

While mood disorders have strong ties to chemical imbalance, anxiety disorders have a strong connection with prior trauma. Anxiety comes from a place of excessive worrying and a lack of control over stressful environments. These worrying thoughts are intrusive, hard to get rid of, and often lead to even more worry down the line. Anxiety medication focuses on calming down the fight-or-flight response caused by excessive worrying. On a similar note, eating disorders such as bulimia and anorexia appear more often in people with an underlying anxiety disorder or prior history of trauma. Post-traumatic stress disorder (PTSD) is also a psychiatric condition that stems from previous trauma which could include a natural disaster, a serious accident, a terrorist act, war/combat or rape, or being threatened with death, sexual violence, or serious injury.

Understanding the characteristics of these common disorders can be useful to help identify the symptoms you or someone else might be experiencing. As we learn to live with our mental health disorders or continue to hide them, we may not appear to demonstrate any of the typical symptoms. Such high-functioning anxiety or depression still affects and impairs a person's ability to go about their daily lives. A psychotherapist, Dr. Mayra Mendez, identifies the effects of high-functioning depression: "Depression may inhibit the desire for activity and action, but high-functioning individuals tend to forge ahead in an effort to succeed with goals. The drive to accomplish often sustains action and moves high-functioning individuals toward getting things done." Since they've learned to mask their internal battles with depression and anxiety, high-functioning people seem to be overachievers at face value. It's harder for such people to discuss their symptoms because there often aren't obvious signs to point to.

Ignoring poor mental health inevitably exacerbates the real harm it causes. For some, mental health struggles get in the way of building and maintaining relationships. Difficulties getting out of bed or leaving the house and increased social anxieties, all symptoms of poor mental health, hinder the ability to develop friendships. People who are suffering from mental illness usually have trouble connecting with friends at a time when they need them the most. During my past depressive episodes, I would often stop responding to messages and ignore friends who reached out to check in on me. In these cases, people are likely to alienate themselves from their communities and networks, as social withdrawal is one of the key signs of depression (Soong and Smith, 2014). Untreated mental health also affects work and productivity, interfering with careers and academic endeavors. Because of my depression during college, I remember skipping most of my classes and letting homework pile on for weeks, which only overwhelmed me further.

THE DISCONNECT

Because there is no one direct cause of mental health conditions, it's quite difficult to understand their onset and progression. No two individuals' experiences with mental health will be the same, but that doesn't mean these experiences aren't real or valid. In South Asian households, mental health conditions are often not considered a *real* issue and are readily dismissed. Specifically, many of the cultural factors mentioned earlier in this chapter inhibit mental health concerns from being taken seriously in South Asian households.

First, the preoccupation with keeping family matters private and keeping up appearances deter people from seeking the help they need. Their concerns are usually dismissed under the guise of "saving face" or maintaining a certain family image. As part of the "model minorities" in America, South Asians are accustomed to demonstrating a strong work ethic, high intelligence, and resilience. You have to be "on" all the time. Any mental weakness is a contradiction of their place in society and at odds with their perceived identity. When and if an issue is raised, the predominant fear is someone will find out and "out" you. When Saba,[3] a twenty-three-year-old Pakistani-American, told her mother that her doctor recommended antidepressant medication, her mother's first response was fear. "Your professors are going to find out and they'll grade you down. You can't do that," Saba's mother told her. The fear of tarnishing a reputation often hinders us from taking mental health seriously.

A problem with mental health is understood in black-and-white terms for our immigrant parents: either you're "crazy" or you're not; either someone has cast the evil eye on you or not. For them, mental health doesn't exist on a spectrum as we understand it today. Conditions like anxiety, depression, and even PTSD aren't considered real because they don't present the typical symptoms of "crazy" that tend to be equated with more serious illnesses such as schizophrenia or bipolar disorder.

Even then, the reflex is to minimize symptoms rather than understand them. Pooja, an Indian-American, described how she witnessed doctors and family members alike dismiss her grandmother's severe postpartum depression (PPD) as fake. "She's just pretending because she doesn't want to cook and clean for her family." When we ourselves don't understand our symptoms, the best we can muster up are vague descriptions, as Pooja's grandmother had to: "I don't feel good today." As women, especially, we're taught not to burden others with our problems. Our collectivist culture requires us to put our

---

3 Saba and all my other interviewees' names have been changed to protect their privacy.

needs second, after those of our family and elders. Pooja's grandmother's illness was only ever considered a scapegoat, a mark of her laziness and negligence. Her PPD caused a daughter to grow up without an attentive mother, an insecurity Pooja recalls her mother lamenting.

Ironically, our status as immigrants makes us more predisposed to mental health issues. The immigrant experience is riddled with emotional trauma: uprooting your life to live in an unfamiliar place, separation from family and loved ones, or the need to assimilate to a new environment where you're a minority. The first-generation immigrant experience is also riddled with similar circumstances: growing up torn between two cultures, taking on the burden of immigrant parents, and racism within the Western society we call home. These difficult life experiences and the emotional toll they take are left unaddressed. Other mental health concerns of South Asians include:

- Social isolation and rejection due to immigrant and minority status, not only for adults in the workplace, but for children and young adults in school.
- First generation tension between balancing ethnic cultural values and mainstream Western values.
- Lack of community for stay-at-home spouses and moms who do not speak the language, have limited social contact, and are dependent upon other family members to navigate the outside world (Das and Kemp, 1997).

These experiences are the exact life changes and environmental factors that are the breeding ground for mental health issues. But, due to the cultural stigma on mental health, these issues (along with others) are swept under the rug far too often. It's time now to not only look back under this rug, but to also clean up the messes we've hidden.

As we become more conscious of our reactions to mental health struggles—both our own and others'—we can begin to reduce the stigma. In tandem, a deeper understanding of mental health and its effects will help us recognize how to take better care of our mental health, including knowing when and how to seek help.

Of course, this journey will not be quick, nor will it be easy. What I can tell you, though, is it will most definitely be worthwhile. If not for you today, then for the future generation. We owe it to them to take on the laborious task of normalizing mental health struggles in our communities. If we don't do this now, we risk passing down these same issues (and others) to our children and grandchildren. Many of us are already intimately familiar with the distress of navigating our mental health in a culture that didn't understand it. It would really be a shame if that was all we could pass down.

It's no longer necessary to carry the harmful cultural practices, the anxiety, the depression, nor any other mental health struggle with us as we build the next generation. As first-generation children of immigrants, we're uniquely empowered with the resources and collective wisdom to celebrate our culture while *also* confronting it for its toxicity. We must collectively raise our voices to finally break the stigma that shackled our ancestors who suffered and struggled silently. It's up to us to do better not just for ourselves, but for those who came before us and those who will come after us.

PART TWO:

THE STORIES WE NEVER TOLD

Poster Child
Log Kya Kahenge? | What will people say?
Sandwich Generation
Family Heirlooms
Mardangi | Manhood
Ammi ki Guriya | My Mother's Doll
Pride

Poster Child

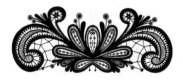

Dear Papa,

Somebody asked me yesterday what my hobbies were. I stared blankly at her face, unable to come up with an answer. "I'm a lawyer," I told her.

"That's not a hobby, it's your job. I mean what do you do for fun?" She said this slower, as if she was trying to translate it for me.

In response, I complained about not having time for hobbies, which seemed a sufficient enough answer for her. I speak English fluently, but "hobby" did sound like a foreign word to me. Do you have a hobby, Papa? Do I have one?

I spent the rest of the day thinking to myself, "What do *I* like to do?" I remembered, suddenly, a conversation we had when I was probably thirteen years old.

I came home ecstatic, waving a piece of paper in the air. I jumped up and down with joy, true and pure joy. I excitedly proclaimed, "I won the art competition! My drawing won the art competition! Can you believe it?"

I shoved my certificate in your face, waiting to see you light up with pride. Three seconds went by. Five seconds. Ten seconds. Fifteen. Your face remained stoic. You mustered a "Good job, *beta*." But even thirteen-year-old Sam could see through your flimsy expression of praise.

You must have had a long day at work. No matter. I went to the kitchen, certificate in hand. Beaming, I carefully placed it on the refrigerator, right at eye-level—impossible to ignore.

After dinner that night, you came to my room. With colored pencils and comic strips scattered on the floor, I was concentrating deeply on drawing my characters in a panel. "*Beta*, what is all of this?" you interrupted.

"I'm making a comic book! I promised Dennis I would show him tomorrow at school." My eyes never left the paper and neither did my pencil.

You cleared your throat. "Listen, Samir." You sat on the bed and motioned for me to join. I had to put my pencil down.

"I need you to understand something, my son. You are growing up now; you're going to be a man very soon. This stuff…" You pointed at my comics. "This stuff is for kids, for girls. *Men* have no business playing with arts and crafts. What will people at the temple say if they saw our son toting a bag full of crayons? This time-wasting bullshit isn't going to support a family—our family."

You went on to say some other things, reminding me I'm the family's "superstar son," that only girls and gays liked art, that I need not waste my time or *your* money on these things. After our conversation, I knew Dennis wasn't going to get his comic book tomorrow. I had a lot of homework to do.

Over time, that conversation repeated itself more frequently and your voice boomed louder.

"You are the only son we have, our only chance," you would say. "We cannot let you squander away the opportunity for greatness to pursue a girls' hobby. You get good grades; you'll get into the best high school in the area, and you'll go to law school. You're going to make us proud in front of the whole community. Your mom and I have always wanted a lawyer in the family, and as our son, it's your responsibility to fulfill those dreams. What else did we come to this country for? Just like you made the tennis team, you'll get into law school and make us proud."

So, my art supply shelf began collecting dust, forgotten, and soon filled with SAT books, then LSAT books.

I became the poster child you always said I was, the patriarch you wanted, the man you said I had to be. Top law school, top grades, top-notch job. Superstar Samir: I am known for excellence, and nothing less. I made you proud, didn't I, Papa? You walk with your head held high, my accomplishments rolling off your tongue at every *davat*.

You've had the answer to all my questions: which school I should go to, which type of law I should practice, which firm I should pick. So tell me, Papa, what are my hobbies? You already told me I couldn't like drawing.

So, do I like golfing, is that the right answer? Do I like boxing? Is that manly enough? Can I like cooking, or is that too girly?

What do I like, Papa?

I guess I should pick a hobby you like. I'm your son; I will likely enjoy what you like to do, right? So I thought back to what you liked to do. I thought long and hard and couldn't find a single thing.

Men like us, we aren't allowed to have hobbies. A Desi man is the provider and the caretaker—nothing else. He doesn't have time for hobbies because there is money to be made and mouths to feed. Weakness isn't an option for the Desi man.

I stayed awake late into the night, asking myself many questions, most of which I didn't have the answer to. I don't know what I like to do. I don't even know what I believe, what I want, or what happiness feels like.

All I do know is I am a poster child, stuck inside the frame on your wall for all to see.

Papa, you wanted me to make you proud, so I did. You wanted me to become a lawyer, so I did. You wanted me to become the leader of this family, so I did. You never asked me what I wanted.

All I wanted is to be less like you and more like me.

Sincerely,
Sam, the lawyer who could have been an artist

The complicated navigation of two cultures often pulls first-generation children of immigrants in opposite directions. While we grow up and assimilate to the American culture around us, we still see the world through the lens of our South Asian heritage—conflict is bound to happen. We're conditioned from a young age not to question the cultural commandments handed to us. Being an immigrant adds a layer of dichotomy to these cultural commandments. There is the way *we* do it and there is the way the *Americans* do it. Whether by coincidence or by intention, the intersection of these two ways of doing things is minuscule. Thus, as first-generation children of immigrants, we often have to pick sides.

As we explore the world around us with access to hobbies, ideas, and ways of thinking that our parents never had, we bring these ideas home. We start forming our identities within these clashing cultures. Sometimes they are welcomed (such as using a Kitchen-Aid to knead dough), other times they are not (having too many friends of the opposite gender). While our parents tend to favor separation of cultures (ours and theirs), South Asian youth tend to integrate these cultures when consolidating our identities. During adolescence, youth encounter many contradictions between their heritage and the host culture, the culture of the country of residence. When conflicting ideals are presented, it is natural that adolescents will take autonomy to pick and choose the ideals they want to live by.

Growing up, children of South Asian immigrant parents often hear phrases like: *That's not acceptable in our culture; We don't do that, we're not American; This is how we have been doing it for generations; That's just the way it is.* We are conditioned to build this separation between ourselves and our friends, classmates, and colleagues. The thought that we're different from them is always in the back of our minds, not one to be celebrated but rather one to be wary of. The "outside world" is posed as dangerous to our way of life—a poison to our culture. And anyone who acts *too American* is immediately deemed the bad apple that's ready to spoil the bunch. Kriti, an Indian-American I interviewed, recounted how her mom often brought up this disparity: "When I was a teenager, and even now, she would say, 'That's so American of you!'" Adopting this American identity, or even parts of it, is not seen as an accomplishment or just another trait. It's seen as a characteristic to be unlearned.

However, the clash of cultures leads parents to believe children have become "corrupted," causing much family conflict. The danger of this possible corruption leads parents to apply extra pressure on children to conform to cultural expectations. Oftentimes parents use the phrase: *haath se nikal gaya/gayi*, meaning the child has gotten out of hand, unable to be kept in check. Parents assume any acculturation with the Western culture means their children are on the "wrong path." Even though questioning traditional values and one's culture is a normal part of adolescence and identity formation, Desi parents tend to take it personally as their own parenting failure (Shariff, 2009). When they feel they have failed to pass down cultural values effectively, they experience parenting stress: conflict or tension within the parent-child dynamic. This tension causes them to react to their children's divergent cultural preferences with anger, increased levels of monitoring and psychological control, and instilling feelings of guilt and shame to redirect their children's behavior (Shariff, 2009).

In this culture that values self-sacrifice, familial and societal expectations are always given more weight than individual desires. If our parents or elders in the family ask us to do something or go somewhere, there's no room for objection. To be deemed an *acha bacha* (or *achi bachi*), a good kid, we must listen to and respect all elders. We are told constantly and consistently our actions represent the family, the race, and the religion—and letting people down is not an option.

Our parents' wishes or desires become instructions—or actually, requirements. Under the guise of parents knowing better, they steer our decisions, likes, dislikes, and beliefs. Of course, parents should guide their children and help them learn right from wrong. There is nothing wrong with parents nudging their children toward liking something they used to enjoy during their childhoods—after all, that's what they know! In fact, studies have shown parental involvement improves academic performance as well as social and cognitive development (Shah, 2015). The tension in South Asian parenting arises when parents' suggestions are actually demands. There was no option for us to reply, "No thanks, I know *you* used to like playing badminton as a kid, but I don't really enjoy it. So, I don't want to be on the team." The response to such a statement usually included guilt, shame, or some combination of the two.

When I was nine years old, my dad finally took my sister and me to Build-A-Bear Workshop (after I begged him for a year). *My own teddy bear I get to design?* I was ecstatic. I ran to the first station and started rummaging through the various bins of unstuffed bears. I ran my fingers through all the furs, making sure my bear's was the softest. Finally, I narrowed it down to two choices. I held them both up and imagined my life with each of the bears by my side. Just then, my dad shoved a third, hideous-looking bear in front of me, "Get this one. It looks nice." I hesitated and looked up at him. I didn't like that bear. I didn't want it. I tried to show him the two bears I was deciding between, but he insisted, ugly bear still shoved in my face. "No, get this one." He handed it to me.

I wanted to say "No," but I truly didn't know how to. So, I took the ugly bear I didn't want and continued my not-so-magical-anymore journey through the workshop. My ugly build-a-bear stayed in its white cardboard house for days after we brought her home. I didn't really ever play with her. She wasn't the buddy I imagined having nor the one I wanted. My dad noticed this neglect and, for months after, he badgered me for begging him to buy me an expensive teddy bear I never played with.

A similar story is Samir's from the beginning of this chapter. Cultural norms that dictate what is acceptable for a boy to enjoy and engage in prevented young Sam from pursuing art, even as a hobby. His father's mandate for him to become a lawyer overtook his own interests or choices. After twenty-eight years, Sam is left with an identity crisis. Growing up under the shadow of his parents' expectations, Sam never had a chance to explore his own identity and personality. He is left questioning the simplest of things: "What are my hobbies?"

As a generation, children of immigrants have struggled with identity crises, losing themselves in the fight between their South Asian heritage and their American nationality. Children who forgo their desires and live the life their parents want are seen as virtuous and exemplary. Hamza, a twenty-nine-year-old Pakistani, recalled learning very early on the "identity [he was] conditioned to have" never felt like his own:

> "From the jump, for any brown kid, whether you're a boy or girl, your life is not your own. You're really unsure where you begin and where your parents' or family's version of you stops."

These identity crises and our ways of coping with them have a larger effect on our mental health. One study found "South Asian youths facing identity conflicts have reported delinquent behavior, alienation from family members, stress, and depression" (Shariff, 2009). Desi kids only get around to exploring our own identities well into our twenties, or when we're physically able to move away (for college or when moving for a job). The freedom and space to find out what *we* like to do and what makes *us* happy is usually not afforded to us initially—we have to consciously seek it and sometimes even fight for it. Sadly, making that intentional choice isn't an option for everyone. Many of us don't even realize what we're missing, and those who do don't know how to make it happen. The fight for that freedom can sometimes cost us our relationships with our families or with our own selves— neither of which we should have to choose between or lose.

The inability to express beliefs, ideas, and interests that might differ from the cultural norm or status quo leads some of us to create double lives for ourselves. The stereotype of an Aisha (or any other Desi teenage girl) swapping her jeans for a miniskirt in the bathroom before school is not the butt of a joke, it's a cry for help. Aisha just wants to wear a mini-skirt, but doing so requires her to hide it from her family. We're forced to do the things we want to do in secret, devising complicated (and creative) plans for small moments of self-expression.

In doing so, sometimes we spring so far away from the shackles of overprotection that we land on the opposite side of the spectrum. It's freedom like we've never seen it before, and we often don't know what do to with it. We check every forbidden item on the list, chickens with our heads cut off, running around with a desperate desire to find ourselves.

When we do get some of that freedom and space, we're not always equipped to handle it in a healthy way. Several interviewees describe their college experiences as difficult transitions. "When I first received freedom in college, I went crazy; I was unstoppable," recounted Hamza. Anvi, twenty-six years old, described her binge drinking spells: "To alleviate feelings, I drank heavily. I would drink to get drunk, and I didn't even know why." This newfound freedom was so foreign for some of us that we didn't know our limits. It was hard for us to make choices for ourselves because that was something we rarely had the opportunity to do growing up.

Another Indian-American, Sejal, described to me how her and several of her South Asian friends were sexually assaulted in college:

> *"The problem with having brown parents is when you leave and turn eighteen, you don't know your limits for things. I didn't know what is and is not okay for a boy or girl to do to you. I didn't know what sexual advances were, and I got sexually assaulted in college within my first couple months of going to school and it was by a brown person."*

As we flock to get a taste of everything we weren't allowed to do, we're unprepared because our parents never equipped us for situations they didn't allow us to be in. Navigating acculturation in an American college system, we're rapidly exposed to new ideas, beliefs, and ways of life neither us nor our parents are accustomed do. We can't go to them for advice. That would only lead to trouble. So, we're left without proper guidance in our double lives.

Upon gaining freedom in college, we also begin to question the authenticity of our actions and beliefs—*Was this me? Or is this my parents?* I don't think I truly came into my own personality until after my first few years of college. Prior to that, I was often a reflection of my parents' beliefs and ideals. I did what I was told without questioning any of it. When I had to start navigating my life by myself, I felt lost. *What do I put on my Subway sandwich? What are people even supposed to do on weekends?* I had no idea. All my Subway sandwiches and weekend plans had always been decided for me.

In fighting this battle with ourselves, our parents, and society, we suffer. Through her qualitative study on South Asians acculturation, Edith Samuel noted, "The process of searching for an identity places [South Asian immigrants] in a state of confusion and conflict" (2005). We begin to question our worth. Our issues with identity can cause low self-esteem and low self-efficacy (i.e., "how effective and in control of their lives people believe they can be"). Since our identity and self-esteem are "interdependent and mutually reinforcing, both a low sense of self-worth and self-efficacy can lead to depressive disorders" (Luyckx et al, 2012). Samuel also found participants "expressed depressive feelings of angst, stress, moodiness, anxiety, loneliness, and trauma as they were subjected to the process of adjustment into the settler society" (2005). When we experience these feelings, getting help is not always an option. The South Asian stigma around mental health issues prevents many of us from seeking help, further worsening these symptoms. What we are left with is a recursive loop of identity crisis and depression.

Our parents came to this country for a better life—a different life. We Desis should be more open to the changes and differences that come with that life. Samir should be able to pursue his artistic passion and still make his parents proud. Aisha's miniskirt shouldn't negate her love for her culture. We're just trying to express and be ourselves. We should be able to freely live a life we get to choose, not one that's forced upon us. We should be given the space and opportunity to develop our identities for our parents to see the real us. There are real people behind the poster children our parents showcase on their walls. They deserve a chance to get to know themselves and be themselves.

Let us out of the posters, please.

Log Kya Kahenge? | What Will People Say?

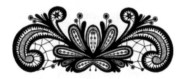

Dear *Log,*

I can't do this anymore. I'm tired of constantly losing this rigged game where you always get to be right. You have a seat at the table in my house—in every house. Your voice is given more weight than mine; I am seldom allowed to speak. Why do you get to control what goes on inside the four walls of *my* house? It seems as though your satisfaction matters more around here than my happiness, than my peace. So, when I cried for help, she didn't ask what I needed, but instead she asked about you.

"*Log kya kahenge?*" my mother said. "A divorce! You can't do that to us, Priya!" *As if I told him to give me that black eye.*

"I can't live like this, Mom. I am constantly living in fear that he'll get upset. And when he gets upset, he hurts me." With tears in my eyes, I pleaded for salvation. "Even over little things. If I don't immediately answer the phone or—"

"Then make sure you answer the phone, *beta*," she interrupted. "It's *your* responsibility to make him happy. Your father worked very hard to get this good match for you. Don't say anything, *ghar ki izzat ka sawal hai!* We have a reputation in the community. You cannot get a divorce."

"Ma, I can't sleep at night. I can't eat. I need to get away. Please, help me." She looked away when I begged. Whether out of shame, fear, or pity, I'm not sure.

So once again, my happiness was thrown to the side. For you People. People who might point fingers and scoff. People who might say I must've been a bad wife. People who might spread rumors that I'm lying. People who might label me as the divorcee—never letting me forget. People who weren't there when he hit me the first time, or the second time. People who weren't there when I needed support.

I kept my head down and played the part, continued to let you see the perfect daughter-in-law you all said I had to be. I covered my scars and bruises with makeup (as a courtesy to you) to make sure you couldn't see the pain and suffering underneath, all to make sure I never gave you an opportunity to say something. But you still see everything, and you always have something to say:

No children yet? Why haven't you given him an heir? Are you sure you're being a good daughter-in-law? Bechari, must just be your kismat. *It's your fault. You're not enough. You're doing it wrong.*

You get to control our lives but only for the worse. You see us suffering, suffocating, sinking. You know when we're wronged, but you don't speak up for us. Instead, they wrong us *because* of you.

I'm forced to stay with my abuser for fear People might have something to say. I cannot stand up for myself, otherwise you'll say I brought shame to my family. I cannot seek help, otherwise you'll label me as crazy.

No matter how much I cry to be let out from here, they won't let me out. Your voice is louder than my screams and my family would rather appease you than free me.

Even with all of you watching me, surrounding me, claiming to be my "community," I have nobody. I'm alone and I'm stuck and there's no way out.

I wish it didn't have to be this way. I wish People, you *log*, who are always so quick to talk, were also that quick to help. Would you have saved me then? If the aunties didn't snicker at the word "divorce," would my mother have let me free myself? Would I be met with support and compassion instead of pity and condemnation?

I also wish I was strong enough to withstand the stares and the whispers. Maybe then I could've found a better way to free myself, one that would let me have a happier ending.

But since I'm not, I know there's only one way for me to win the rigged game against you, *log*. Since my bruised lip and black eye weren't enough to call your attention, maybe the sound of a gunshot will be. Maybe that way my voice will be heard. I hope by freeing myself, my mother will finally hear my screams over what other people have to say.

I hope this time, when I pull the trigger, I'm loud enough to save another Priya from feeling as stuck as I did. When you see what you did to me, I hope you think twice about what your words can really do.

At least this time when they ask *log kya kahenge*, I won't hear it.

Sincerely,
Priya, the girl who could have (and should have) been saved

Log kya kahenge? This mantra is etched so deeply into our minds that we don't even need our parents to ask us this question anymore. We do it ourselves. In our culture, our lives are dictated not by us, but rather by what others might think of us. But "*log kya kahenge*" isn't actually the inquiry it appears to be. At best it's a rhetorical question not-so-subtly nudging us to stay in our place. We're reminded there is already an identity and path chosen for us, one we're forbidden from veering away from. (Ironically) There is no question about it.

Our parents (and society) give us an ultimatum based on a certain valued appearance, attitude, and mannerism. *This is the only way to be you. You are who I tell you you are. We know best.* We're suffocated by this proclamation that controls the gears running our society, where everyone is the judge, jury, and executioner. The morality of outsiders is revered no matter how unjust they may be. *Log kya kahenge* is control by another name.

Our society expects (demands) we do things and behave a certain way, and they're not quiet about it. The communities we're a part of are quick to judge our actions and circumstances without even knowing the full story. We're stripped of agency in our own lives. The People run this show and we're merely their puppets. The puppet masters, then, feel entitled to know the goings-on in every household. They've already stripped away our agency, so they take our privacy as well. Under the guise of *log kya kahenge*, the South Asian community around us becomes a sort of Big Brother. As we try to navigate forming an identity, even if in secret, we must watch out for the surveillance from those around us. If we think our parents aren't watching, some aunty definitely is. If we're found to be doing anything other than what is expected of us, we're shamed and guilted about it. We've not only disobeyed our elders, but we have tarnished their reputation of perfection and order.

Under the watchful eye of *log kya kahenge*, we grow up afraid—of our families, of society, and of ourselves. We betray our own identities, opting to be ourselves only in private. Even then, we're cautious. But when we do get to be who we are, it's still with a hint of shame, a grief because we're either lying to our parents or lying to ourselves. While they're quick to reprimand us for veering out of line, we're also rewarded with praise and celebration for being the best at forgoing our own identity to adopt their expectations. This is often the only approval we get; it becomes addicting. So, we seek this approval whenever we can and, in the process, further suffocate our own happiness, desires, and aspirations.

Over time, our approval-seeking behaviors turn into a constant desire and need to please others, often at the cost of our own happiness. We were conditioned to think our worth and value was derived not from our individuality and humanness, but rather how well we could fit into the mold of others' expectations. We're constantly chasing something we'll never reach in hopes to gain approval from our society. But the *log* are never satisfied; they always find something to judge us over.

Collectively, Asian Americans have often been described as a "model minority" due to their above average academic and career success. This model minority concept is often used to talk about race and depicts Asians as the minority group that "made it" in America—the rags to riches story everyone loves to hear. But with this badge of the model minority comes the constant pressure of having to defend it. This stereotype portrays Asian Americans as a hardworking, intelligent, productive, and successful group. From a young age, academic success is drilled into our heads as the only way to achieve the American dream. Our identity and self-validation become correlated to this success. In a *Times* article, Sanjana Sathian recalls her experience: "Having so little vocabulary for selfhood, I and others like me clung to the sole fact we knew about ourselves: we achieved in those arenas like our lives depended on it" (2021).

We're socialized to believe the best way to repay our parents' sacrifices and immigrant struggle is through boundless achievement (Chang, 2017). With this comes immense guilt for not fitting into the mold or for underachieving the community's impossibly high and rigid standards for success. Our fear is not just of the failure, but more so of what others would say about that failure. We wouldn't be able to measure up to the WhatsApp scorecards our parents use to compare our successes. The model minority myth gives the *log* the exact weapon they need to exert control. There's already a blueprint laid out for us; the rules are written. There are a few acceptable professions and paths. Nothing else is good enough.

As we strive for perfection, we end up sacrificing our own wellbeing for our family's desires and image. We overwork and overexert ourselves to achieve dreams that aren't even ours, all to make sure the family reputation and others' opinions can be maintained. Because of our model minority status, attention is only paid to academic and professional success. Other achievements often don't count or garner the same respect and adoration as getting into any Ivy League would. For those of us who are pursuing interests in the arts or nontraditional fields, our achievements (even if they are remarkable) are never appreciated or accepted with the same pride. If it cannot be bragged about and equated to the narrow definition of success engrained in our community, it's not worthy.

This negatively impacts mental health, as we begin to tie our self-worth to an often unattainable and unrealistic ideal. Our people-pleasing makes it difficult for us to stand up for ourselves and, consequently, we tend to have lower self-esteem. Many first-generation children find it difficult to be authentic to who they are. We end up living double lives—one for parents and one for ourselves. But even with our double life comes the anxiety of being found out for who we *truly* are, and the consequent wrath of what others will say. Even living double lives, we find ourselves alone. Having to constantly hide part of who we are, we're seldom able to seek the support we want and need from our parents. For example, those who need to keep their dating lives a secret from their families aren't allowed the space to grieve a breakup or freely talk through relationship problems. Because they can't reveal why they might be upset or struggling, they must pretend it doesn't exist. On top of having trouble standing up for themselves, not having the support of their families makes it difficult for some to leave toxic relationships, pushing them further into isolation.

In pursuit of perfectionism, Desi society chooses only to value what is positive; everything else is swept under the rug. We don't talk about difficult things—not as families, and not as a society. Big Brother is watching and if we talk about something negative, he will hear us. So, we keep silent. This is especially problematic when it comes to mental health. When, and if, children seek support from their parents regarding their mental health, they're shut down by *log kya kahenge.* There is a fear of shattering the perfectly curated image that "everything is fine." An Indian-American, Dev, described how even though his parents let his brother seek therapy, "they didn't want their friends to know what was happening." There's also a fear of telling someone else something negative about you, something that might tarnish your reputation if it came out. So, seeking help or therapy for a mental health concern becomes out of the question. "Why would we want someone else to know our business? You can talk to us about your problem," they say. But we can't.

When we're struggling with something they *can't* know about, how are we going to talk to them about our problems? Before (and if) the issue at hand would even be discussed, we'd first get in trouble for being in a situation we weren't supposed to be in. Sri Lankan-American Anvi remembers telling her parents, "Nothing made me think I could come to you with my problems," when they asked why she hadn't told them about being sexually assaulted when it happened. Anvi knew she'd be met with a barrage of questions and "I told you so's" if she had opened up to them. "They would get mad at me for drinking or partying. Our conversation wouldn't actually be constructive," Anvi said.

At its worst, this obsession with others' opinions can even lead to disownment. Some families would rather sever all ties with their children who "have gone astray" than accept the nontraditional decisions they made. Travel blogger Disha Smith's family disowned her because she chose to be with someone of a different race and religious background. For

Disha, *log kya kahenge* literally tore her family apart. When her parents found out about her relationship:

> "*I received an angry call from my mom. She called me every degrading name in the dictionary and said I was the biggest screwup she had ever met. She said I was ruining our family name in the Indian society they were a part of. [My father] said I was a disgrace to the family and he was ashamed about what he was going to tell his friends and society about me dating Amos. I begged him to meet Amos, but he was not interested in doing so. He never cared how I felt or what I wanted—the only thing he cared about was his reputation*" (Smith, 2019).

Disha described how her parents then had her followed and attempted to kidnap her to ensure her relationship would not continue:

> "*My parents said I needed to move back home and I would be under twenty-four seven supervision once I moved back. They said they would make sure I had no access to the outside world and they would get me married to some random stranger within a few months. They even started listing off names of prospects*" (Smith, 2019).

They eventually gave her an ultimatum—them or him.

While Disha's case seems extreme, it does still happen in this day and age. She was able to utilize her resources to keep herself safe and escape this toxic situation, but not everyone is as lucky (though she still lost her family in the process).

The obsession with reputation imposes conditionality on Desi families' love for their children. If you follow the mold, you're the poster child. If not, you're unworthy of love and respect. To put that burden on a child (or anyone for that matter) is not just unfair, it's wrong!

Hungry for others' approval, our parents and families emotionally abuse us into submission. We're forced to make choices to appease them, to save face and save our relationship with them. We shouldn't have to choose between our family and our own wellbeing, but Desis are often put in that position by their loved ones.

As in Priya's case from the beginning of this chapter, we're told to suck it up if things aren't as picture-perfect as they seem. If these problems aren't addressed, they don't exist, right? Families will often look the other way and feign ignorance or remain in silent complacency so as not to reveal or acknowledge there might be a problem. What's worse: your child being abused by their spouse, or others finding out your child is being abused by their spouse?

Out of fear of what others will say, families will minimize and dismiss mental health concerns. In protecting their image, they fail to protect their children. Mental health is ignored until it can't be, when it's too late, like it was for Priya. After begging to be protected from her situation, Priya felt alone and helpless. Many, like Priya, have made the difficult decision of taking their lives because they felt trapped on all ends. They were trapped by a family they couldn't go to about a situation they weren't allowed to get out of.

Priya could have been saved if our lives weren't dictated by *log kya kahenge.* If saving face was less important than saving a child from an abusive marriage, she could have been saved. If People are going to talk, could they at least talk about something that is going to help us rather than hurt us?

Sandwich Generation

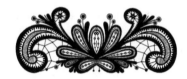

Dear *Dada,*

I think I've finally made it. I have been chasing this so-called "American dream" for twenty years now. I know you would be proud of the life I created here. It's a bit different from home—the fruit isn't as sweet, and the colors don't ever shine as bright as they do back home. but it's what I was able to build here, bit by bit, scrap by scrap.

I often think about the home I left behind. But my memories of playing cricket in the street with my brothers and carrying home *sabzis* with you from the market down the street are fading. With every passing day, the boy with the cricket *balla* in his hand becomes a stranger to me. I may have achieved his hopes and dreams, but I've forgotten why he wanted all of that in the first place.

That boy came with me to America in search of something better. But sometime during the pursuit of this American dream, he left. When *daal chawal* was replaced by lasagna and cricket was replaced by football, he left. When daily phone calls to you and *Dadi* were replaced by late nights at the office, he left.

In his stead, he left me in charge. I think I've done a pretty good job, though I wonder if he would be impressed.

Yesterday, *Abu* came to me, very upset. *Dada*, I'm not one to complain, but I'm not sure who was right and who was wrong. What do you think?

"I've been telling you for a week now, Ansar, my iPad is not working right! How is your mother supposed to watch her dramas and how am I supposed to check my Facebook messages? This is the third time I have told you, *beta*." Was my sixty-eight-year-old father scolding me?

"I'm sorry, *Abu*, I've been dealing with a lot of deadlines at work. I haven't had a chance to take a look." I tried to buy myself some more time. "Have you asked Haris? He's better at this technology stuff anyways. I'm sure he'll be able to fix it in no time."

"Pfft." He scoffed. "Haris never has any time for us. He's always out of the house, doing God knows what. What kind of an American boy are you raising? Back home, we stayed home to help our parents." *Abu*'s favorite line. *Dada*, was *Abu* actually always home when he was younger, or does he just like to bring that up to make us feel bad?

"Haris goes to work, *Abu*. He has a job so he can save up for college. I'll ask him when he comes home tonight to help you fix your iPad. Otherwise, I'll look at it when I come back home tonight after dinner," I told him reassuringly.

"Where are you going?" He seemed more offended than curious.

"Well, I wanted to take Shazia out to dinner. We haven't been out, just the two of us, in a long, long time. But don't worry, *Abu*. Shazia already made *sabzi* for you and *Amma* to eat. It's all ready to go on the stove. She made fresh *rotis* for you too. She knows how much you like those." Why did I feel like I was still going to be in trouble?

"I guess there's nothing more than *sabzi* and *roti* in your mother and I's *kismat**. You would think once we were in America our son would treat us to something more than the poor man's dinner. I guess you guys have become more American than Indian now. Besides, why would you take us anywhere..." His voice trailed off and he mumbled something under his breath. I lowered my gaze, unable look him in the eyes. I didn't have any words to reply to his accusations with anyway.

Dada, please tell me. Who is right and who is wrong?

I spent the last twenty years building a life I thought *Abu* would be proud of, that he should be proud of. I spent the last twenty years trying to make sure he would never lift another finger. And he doesn't. Is going to dinner without them really such a slap in the face? Am I wrong to take a break for myself? For Shazia?

I thought when I brought them here, they would get to learn all the things we didn't have the chance to learn. The things I couldn't learn, because survival was our priority. Do you remember, *Dada*, how I always wanted to learn how to play the piano? I was always fascinated by the black and white keys of Rafiq *chachu's* dusty old keyboard, tinkering with them any chance I got. Despite its two missing keys, that piano filled the room with serenity whenever Rafiq *chachu* touched it. I would spend hours listening to him play, mimicking his fingers on my own imaginary piano.

When I could finally afford it, a piano was the first thing I bought, along with piano lessons. For Haris. If I never learned to play the piano, at least my son could play it for me. I was so excited to hear that familiar sound fill the room again. But Haris quit those lessons within weeks, leaving another piano covered in dust. "The piano just isn't *me*. I'd rather learn how to play the guitar," he told me.

For twenty years, our only priority was to survive. Shazia and I did everything we could so they wouldn't have to lift a finger, so we could pay them back for raising us. We did everything we could so our children could live a life better than ours. We broke our backs, hands, and hearts working as hard as we could. We accomplished what we set out to do. But it never seems like it's enough. They always want more, but I'm not sure we have anything left to give.

Dada, I'm not one to complain, but I think I have become sandwiched. My wife and I, we are sandwiched between these two generations. We spent our lives making sure our children had everything we never had and our parents could finally have everything they never could give us. In between them, we have been squeezed out of the picture. In living for them, we didn't get to live for ourselves.

I know I'm proud of the life I've created for my family. But I'm not sure I'm proud of the life I lived myself. At the end of the day, I no longer belong to the home I left, nor do I belong to the home I created. I'm merely a bridge, over which my family was able to build their life. Did you ever feel this way, *Dada*? Surrounded by family, goals accomplished, yet still not able to feel whole? I'm not sure the boy with the cricket *balla* would be impressed with how I ended up. All he really wanted was for me to be happy, to live a life rich in experiences. And that's the only thing I didn't get to do.

Someone once told me: "*apne budhe baap ko nahi bhoolna*" or "*don't forget about your aging father.*" In making sure to never forget my parents, their sacrifices, their needs and wants, I forgot myself. Now that I am almost a *budha baap*, are they going to forget me?

Sincerely,
Ansar, of the Sandwich Generation

We've all heard our parents' coming-to-America stories. They were young with barely any money in their pockets. Some of them were newlyweds, two strangers arriving to an even stranger land. In seeking a better life, our parents left everything they knew: their country, their family, their home. With the excitement of a new place and the promise of a better future also came a scary reality: having left everything and everyone they knew, our parents had to build everything from the ground up.

Packed in between the *handis* and *sarees*, they also brought with them the culture and traditions from the home they left behind. The home that, twenty years later, doesn't look, sound, or even smell the same. Over time, their customs became commandments because those were the only roadmaps they brought. Within them, the burdens and traumas passed down from generations made their way to America too. Our parents clung onto them because these roadmaps were what made their new houses feel like home. This was the way they knew how to live. In times of crisis and hardship, they always went back to what they knew, the frayed, familiar pages filled with wisdom and folly alike. But not every page in this playbook is penned with *Nani's totkas*. Some pages are etched with ancestral toxicity, complacently passed down by our *buzurks*. The patriarchal norms and expectations of self-sacrifice are well-preserved, passed down whether we wanted them or not.

In these foreign lands, our parents sought to bring as much familiarity as they could. Along with building families, they built communities through which they could preserve their culture and pass it down to future generations. These constructed communities replicated what they left back home and became their escape. The brotherhood they couldn't get from Steve at the office, they found from Sanjeev at the temple. A community to rely on can be a healthy coping mechanism. But it can also become a destructive, unhealthy, and addictive fixation. With no one else to go to, the proxy families created here gave the immigrant generation unhealthy ways to cope with their hardships. *Davats* and *kitty parties* were on the calendar every weekend until 2:00 a.m., like clockwork. If someone invited you, you had to go, whether you wanted to or not. There was, of course, delicious homecooked food and comfortable, familiar clothing at these *davats*; all the *biryani* and *korma* you were craving during the week. But these communities were also filled with gossiping aunties, parents comparing their children, their cars, the sizes of their houses. Constant competition brewing under a façade of kinship. These bonds were only strong when it came to sharing recipes and clothes—never vulnerabilities.

Any struggle or difficulty our parents faced as they rebuilt their uprooted lives went unchecked. They didn't have any mental health support for themselves, nor were they willing or able to seek it out. They had to pay the bills, raise the kids, support the parents, learn the language, navigate the bureaucracy, and send money back home to those they left behind. Survival was the only thing on their minds. Addressing mental health challenges wasn't something they knew how do, nor was it something they thought was necessary. Saba, a Pakistani-American, remembered how her mom reacted when she mentioned her mental health: "I told her I didn't feel good and wanted to see a therapist, and she replied with, 'I haven't been feeling good for twenty years, that's just how it is.'" Even though she may have been struggling with it herself, Saba's mom dismissed mental health altogether and never sought help. Arup, a Bengali-American, learned growing up, "If your life sucks, you just live with it. It's celebrated that you're living a sucky life."

Our parents internalized their feelings of isolation and loneliness, unable and unwilling to share them with anyone. To them, this was just part of the immigrant package. Out of fear of judgment and shame, they didn't share these struggles with their community or even with their families back home. They were living out the precious American dream—at least that's what they had to project.

So as the children of immigrants, we became their therapists. I often hear first-generation children "grew up too quickly." What is really happening behind the scenes is known as parentification: a role reversal between the parents and children where children have to parent their parents. Examples include mediating family conflicts, being an emotional support for the parent, and responsibilities (not chores) to maintain the home (Preciado, 2020). There are two types of parentification and, in immigrant households, we see both at play.

Emotional parentification refers to when the child provides emotional support for their parents: "the emotional tasks assigned to a child may include serving as a confidant for the parent, being entrusted with sensitive information that is developmentally inappropriate (e.g., financial hardship, marital discord), mediating family conflicts, and taking on the role of peacekeeper" (Preciado, 2020). In instrumental parentification, children perform essential functional tasks to maintain the household including cooking, cleaning, providing financial support, taking care of paperwork, and providing care for their siblings. Sometimes these tasks are necessary in immigrant households where parents lack the generational knowledge and wealth required to navigate the "American dream." This is a part of the immigrant experience. Even as a third grader, I gladly wrote business e-mails for my dad (they made me feel so adult). Who else would do it? It would be wrong, though, to ignore the consequences of spending a childhood feeling responsible for such completing such tasks: I grew up too quickly. Without realizing it, I was robbed of a carefree and innocent childhood.

This especially rings true for the eldest child, who likely serves as the third parent for their siblings and sometimes even a pseudo-spouse for their parents. From a young age, eldest daughters might have to fill in the role of a mother and a wife, cooking and cleaning for their siblings and father (who probably seldom set foot in the kitchen). This heavy responsibility causes many firstborns to struggle with their mental health, as they're more likely to experience depression. Child psychologist Dr. Rachel Andrew confirms "as the eldest, being given responsibility constantly can see the child having more in common with adults rather than their peers. They can also internalize that in order to be loved/ accepted, they need to work hard and be responsible. These patterns can lead to depression in adolescence/adulthood, particularly if in spite of working hard, success does not seem to be achieved" (Love, 2014).

Assuming the role of the third parent, eldest children are assumed to be the primary decision-maker on behalf of the family, especially in immigrant households. We're celebrated as independent but, in many cases, that trait was born out of the responsibility to take care of the family at home and outside. The firstborn is the translator, the ambassador to the outside world. This forces many of us to be the peacekeepers in the family, trying to juggle conflicts between parents or siblings. As adults, we firstborns continue this pattern as people-pleasers. We often don't know how to advocate for ourselves because we spent our childhoods advocating on behalf of our parents to our siblings or on behalf of our siblings to our parents.

Emotional parentification is much more complicated because it directly and negatively affects children's social and emotional development. Preciado reminds us that "a child who continuously provides for others—particularly at the expense of themselves—is likely to experience insecure attachments and feelings of unworthiness" (2020). Studies have also linked emotional parentification to higher levels of depression and loneliness (Hooper et al, 2015). Children of immigrants become parentified when serving as pseudo-therapists for their parents to unload the emotional burdens of living and raising children in a foreign country. This excessive emotional caretaking, at an age where we're developmentally unprepared, reinforces placing our needs secondary to others' needs. When we grow up, we find it difficult to maintain healthy boundaries in our relationships. We grew up with blurred boundaries; the pattern is set to be repeated. Blurred boundaries also lead to enmeshment trauma where "everybody's identities, feelings, needs, and expectations are bleeding into each other" (Ahluwalia, 2020). Feeling our parents' heavy burdens as children is often far too much for us to process properly.

Family enmeshment exists because of codependency in relationships, which is deeply rooted in South Asian families since selflessness and sacrifice, especially for elders, is expected. According to Dr. Nicole LePera, clinical psychologist, "Codependency is a learned behavior that begins in childhood, when there's a lack of boundaries within our family dynamic. We learn as children that in order to receive love, we have to be hypervigilant to the emotional state of others around us" (2019). This codependency is apparent when parents depend so heavily on their children for emotional support that neither person has a sense of being nor functioning as their own independent person. Krish, an Indian-American, described the lack of boundaries between his sister and mother: "She was with her twenty-four seven. As the daughter, she was the listening ear all the time." Krish's mother depended heavily on his sister for emotional support, and she wasn't able to be her own person.

Enmeshment and codependency in relationships also breeds a desire to appease and fulfill other people's high expectations. Most of these outcomes affect children well into adulthood, as they become engrained with these habits growing up. As adults, South Asian children may find it difficult to make decisions for themselves because family members have usually taken it upon themselves to do that for them based on their expectations.

We're not only our parents' therapists—we're also the center of their worlds. As Samir's story reminded us from "Poster Child," immigrant parents typically don't have hobbies. So, *we* become their hobbies; their kids are their pride and joy and they devote all their time, money, and energy into them. We become their emotional support *and* their social support. My mom has often told me that she doesn't need to hang out with friends or try out hobbies because: "You guys are enough for me." While that made me feel special, I also found it unfair. Our parents restrict themselves from expressing or exploring their own identities and interests for their families. Ansar, from our story, found himself constantly appeasing either his parents or his children throughout his life. He felt pressured by high expectations and derived his sense of purpose from taking care of others, putting his own needs second. When he planned a date with his wife as an attempt to prioritize himself, he felt guilty. Another immigrant father, fifty-eight-year-old Vijay, told me how stuck he felt throughout his life:

> "We're required to spend resources on everyone except ourselves. I could never afford to withdraw for it. I couldn't just go on vacation and leave them behind. I would feel guilty for not taking my parents with me everywhere. There is guilt all the time in this generation."

In a foreign land, our parents raised us with the familiar ideals they brought along. More often than not, these ideals are what make us who we are today—the proud, third-culture children of immigrants. Sometimes these ideals and the immigrant experience together create circumstances that created trauma for both our parents and us. In prioritizing survival, our parents neglected their own emotional needs. And as they raised children while trying to cope with a lack of emotional support, much of their trauma passed down to us. We see this in mothers lamenting their marriage woes to their daughters. Twenty-four-year-old Aarti described her fear of getting married seeing her parents' marriage as an example: "I saw my mom pride herself on staying with my dad in a marriage without any love. This is what I thought marriage was supposed to be and I definitely didn't want that." We see this in fathers internalizing their struggles, remaining distant from their children, and focusing only on providing for their family.

The homes that were once our parents' don't exist anymore. And the homes that are now theirs never really felt like their own to begin with. Between what was and what sort of is, our parents are sandwiched. They lose a lot of who they were but find it difficult to seek help. So, their unresolved traumas and learned codependent behaviors are passed down to us. As the first generation, we are grateful for everything our parents did for us, but we are allowed to acknowledge the pain they caused. And while we can only wish things were different for us and for them, we can do the work now to make sure this cycle doesn't repeat itself when we parent the future generation.

Family Heirlooms

Dear Ma,

Children aren't meant to carry fragile items. Didn't you know? They're not meant to carry heavy loads. Yet, you tossed that family heirloom into my hands with such reckless abandon. Isn't that child endangerment?

Our family heirloom: honor, *izzat*. A generations-old stone, you told me it holds our ancestors' truths (and also their lies). It turns out when you hand this stone to a daughter, it turns into glass. Fragile glass, waiting for even the faintest of whiffs to cause a crack.

Why are you playing in the sun? Your skin will get dark. Crack. *Why did you get your period so early? Now you're a liability.* Crack. *Why did Sanjana get a better grade than you?* Crack.

Why aren't you praying? Crack. *Why did your father yell at me? What did you do?* Crack. *Why was that boy talking to you? Is he your boyfriend?* Crack. *That top makes you look like a whore. Why are you trying to get attention?* Crack. *Why do you laugh so loudly?* Crack. *Why are you sitting like a boy? Close your legs.* Crack. *Why are you playing in the sun? Your skin is getting dark.* Crack. *Why did you get your period so early? Now you're a liability.* Crack. *Why did Sanjana get a better grade than you?* Crack. *Why aren't you praying?* Crack.

Crack.
Crack.

The cracks keep forming, each poking a new shard of fragile ancestral glass into my back as I carry the burden of our family's honor. Each poke leaves a scar. Scars that I live with, scars that I cannot hide anymore. Some of them still hurt, some of them are merely visual reminders of the burden I am destined to carry. But, why am I telling you all this? You're already familiar with the damage this *izzat* causes. You must have scars of your own.

If it is a mother's duty to protect her children, how come you did not protect me from this heirloom? If you have scars of your own, why did would you hand me the same burden to carry?

If you knew my happiness would be at odds with taking care of this family's honor, why did you take that chance at happiness from me? My destiny is confined to the four walls of our house—because the *izzat* must be protected. My every move watched with so much fear, fear that this family heirloom might become damaged. What was the point of having a daughter when the *izzat* was going to be at risk with every breath she took?

Yet, I did my best to protect this *izzat*. I fulfilled the duty with grace. I came home when I was supposed to, I wore what I was supposed to, I spoke only to who I was supposed to. All to protect this fragile family heirloom I didn't ask for.

I did everything right, mended each crack as it formed. Just how you taught me. But, you didn't mention that no matter how much I try to take care of this *izzat*, it would still be stolen from my hands in the blink of an eye.

I was at the library, exactly where I said I would be. Studying, doing exactly what I said I would be doing. I was wearing jeans and a baggy sweatshirt, comfy studying clothes, exactly what I left home wearing. He looked over at me and smiled. *Surely an innocent smile back would not hurt my izzat.* I smiled back. I continued to concentrate on my *Introduction to Marketing* textbook, taking notes on my computer. I could feel his eyes staring intently at me. Occasionally, I looked up, feigning to look for the iced coffee that was sitting next to my laptop so I could confirm my suspicions. We locked eyes for a split second, but I quickly turned my head back down toward my book. *Don't forget about the izzat.*

A while later I got up to refill my water bottle. As I was waiting at the water fountain, someone tapped my shoulder. It was him. "Excuse me, hi. Sorry to bother you like this."

Dumbfounded, I mustered nothing more than an "Ummm..."

"I don't mean to be so forward, but you're really cute. I've seen you study here a couple times, but I've never had the courage to say anything until now."

"Oh, thank you. That's really sweet of you." I smiled politely. *Is that what I'm supposed to say?*

"Well actually, I was wondering if you wanted to hang out sometime? Maybe get some coffee or a drink or something or whatever…"

Don't forget about the izzat. I stopped him mid-sentence. "Actually, I don't think I'm interested. I'm sorry. I don't really have time to date anyone." My go-to response.

"It's just one date, c'mon," he replied, a bit irritated.

"Look, I'm sorry, but like I said, I don't really have time to date. I'm not interested in going on a date." *Don't forget about the izzat.* I grabbed my overflowing water bottle from the bottle filler.

"Fine. Suit yourself, bitch." He huffed and stomped away, turning a few heads in the quiet library.

As I walked back to my table, I looked outside and realized it was about to get dark soon; that meant I needed to be home. I collected my things and packed up my bag. I got up and made my way toward the lobby.

Footsteps shuffled quickly behind me as I exited the building. "Hey! Excuse me!" he yelled behind me. *Maybe I left something behind on the table.* I stopped and turned around.

"Hi…Uh…Sorry about earlier. Didn't mean to burst out at you like that. Are you sure you don't want to go and just grab a coffee? There's a place nearby that's really cool." He was very persistent.

"Ohhh…No, thank you, I actually need to get home." I tried to be as polite as I could, but now I was getting annoyed. *Don't forget about the izzat.*

He grabbed my hand. "C'mon, please. You're really beautiful." I tried to twist my hand out of his strong grip.

"Please let go of my hand." He got closer, towering over me, as I struggled to free my hand from his ironclad hold. *Don't forget about the izzat.*

"No." Suddenly, he grabbed my waist and pushed himself against my body. I didn't even realize when or how he pinned my hands behind me, but he did. He threw his lips on mine. I closed my eyes and tried to bite down as hard as I could. That only turned him on more.

I did everything I could to protect it. But he took it from me. Shattered it into a million pieces. The *izzat* I protected with every ounce of my being, a stranger came and took it. Why does he get to take something that was never his to begin with? Something I didn't even offer him.

I'm left asking, Ma, will people still value me now that the *izzat* is gone? What's the price I have to pay for protecting my *izzat*?

Sincerely,
Nisha, the daughter who did everything right but still couldn't do anything right

Honor, *izzat*, is the lens through which many South Asians navigate their realities. It's the highly valuable currency via which status and identity is maintained within our communities. As it's earned, this badge of honor is worn proudly by the men in the family, their heads held high. But the burden of protecting and guarding this honor is placed solely on the women in society, especially daughters. The *izzat* of a family is almost entirely dependent on the actions and reputation of the women in the family.

Izzat is a *lathi* used to shepherd women and girls to follow patriarchal, societal expectations. Under the guise of family honor, girls are required to maintain a "sober," timid demeanor, to be the "good" daughters. Their behavior is governed in order to ensure their purity and innocence (and virginity). Men and boys are seldom required to bear the responsibility of the family honor with such severe austerity. Even when they do, men lose honor over the fact that they failed to *control the women* in their family rather than for their own mistakes, which are usually overlooked or minimized. A man's honor is only his, but a woman's honor tarnishes the reputation of entire families. In part of an ethnographic study on South Asian youth, eighteen-year-old Mona described why her family's reputation dissuaded her from dating:

> "*Although I have been approached, yes, it is my, uh, choice because I just don't want to face the consequences, like, why put myself through that trouble... my parents would be very disappointed and I just don't want to put them through that...also because my, um, my uncle's kind of big in society, the Tamil society...so then if I do something wrong, his name kind of gets ruined...and then, um, that reflects bad on our church*'" (Zaidi et al, 2016).

The notion of family honor is so deeply connected to women that the euphemism for rape is: "*izzat lut gaye hai*," meaning "your honor has been robbed." And because the family *izzat* is always at stake, daughters are considered a liability. There are many stories of parents burying newborn daughters alive, their death more preferable than the liability of raising them. In South Asia, sex-selective abortions are common. One study estimated over one hundred thousand abortions of female fetuses during the late 1990s in India (Arnold et al, 2002). If a girl is born, condolences are offered—"Next time it will be a boy"—but if it's a son, then "it's a blessing." As the eldest of three daughters, I'm no stranger to pitying looks from people as they bemoan, "No boys? Only girls?"

A daughter's every move is surveilled with scrutiny by parents, family members, and even the wider community. For women, safeguarding the family's *izzat* requires modesty, chastity, and conformity to the rules prescribed by the patriarchal family leaders. When honor has been lost, restoring it is often done with extreme measures. This phenomenon is specifically known as honor violence, which can include "social isolation, psychological and physical mistreatment, domestic violence, forced suicide, forced marriage, marital rape, and even murder [honor killings]" (Christianson et al, 2021).

Honor-related violence is not only commonplace in much of South Asia, it is also seldom reported or prosecuted. These tactics are often socially acceptable and deemed as appropriate responses to the perceived loss of honor. Male leaders of the family take it upon themselves to restore honor by committing and admitting to honor killings. Recently, a father in India was arrested as he walked to the police station holding the decapitated head of his daughter. He beheaded his own daughter over a relationship he did not approve of (CBS, 2021). Other victims have been attacked with acid and even burned alive because of honor-related violence. A daughter wearing revealing clothes or merely talking to a boy will tarnish the family reputation, but murder and violence against women isn't considered a threat to a family's honor? It seems these are badges barbaric men wear with pride, corpse in hand.

To protect their *izzat*, families impose strict rules on their children, especially their daughters. These rules look different for immigrants than they would have back home, but the goal remains the same: control. On the offensive, parents use shame and guilt to coerce their children into submission. It's considered shameful to not follow the strict norms and values that are in place to supposedly protect us. From a young age, we're painted a picture of what not to do, cautioned against becoming the women who ruin their family's honor and are exiled for it. The gift of family, community, and love is conditional and only for those who can manage to protect their *izzat*. The cautionary tales of women who failed to protect their family's honor were our bedtime stories—we knew the drill. As Sumaiya Ahmed describes, we're given only one roadmap on how to protect this honor:

> *"I'd always been brought up to believe the only way to live a good and happy life was to do everything I possibly can, and more, to make my parents happy. To make them proud. To not ruin their izzat: their reputation, their honor, their name. I was raised with the belief that if I ever became anything than what my parents wanted me to be, or did anything they didn't deem right, then I would shame not just myself, but my father, too"* (Ahmed, 2020).

As daughters, we carry this heavy family heirloom on our backs in a world that doesn't make it easy. Even when we do everything right, as Nisha did, we are told we didn't do enough. There's no winning when every breath you take is meticulously scrutinized. It's as if they want us to fail, like they're looking for any excuse to blame us for betraying the family.

We're always burdened with immense guilt and constant fear that any error we make will be the one that tarnishes the family honor, the one that they make examples of.

Guilt is a conditioned emotion that we learned to feel based on our culture and upbringing. At times guilt can be constructive, serving as the north star to our moral code. But when guilt is used to manipulate and control others' behaviors, it becomes toxic. Therapist John Kim notes "more often than not, instead of bringing about growth, success, and achievement, guilt often brings discouragement, feelings of inferiority, and potentially a whole host of psychological issues" (Kim, 2020). Evoking feelings of inadequacy and self-doubt, excessive guilt begets shame.

Dr. Brené Brown describes guilt as a behavior, a moment in time where our judgment has lapsed, but shame is linked to our self-image, "something we've experienced, done, or failed to do makes us unworthy" (Brown, 2013). Guilt leaves us feeling some control over our behavior. With shame, we feel as if this is something we cannot control—our deviancy is who we are. As soon as guilt becomes shame, it becomes toxic and affects our self-perception. Constantly being made to feel shame about our actions, we become conditioned to believe we *are* the pariahs that our parents warned us not to be.

In South Asian culture, parents often use guilt and shame to manipulate and mold their children's behaviors. One of the most prevalent "guilt trips" used by parents is to weaponize the sacrifices they made to immigrate and build a life in a foreign country for their children's future. Our parents' sacrifices are thrown in our faces whenever they don't approve of our decisions. "How could we not appreciate it?" they ask. But we do. The sacrifices they made aren't lost on us. We recognize and are grateful for the hurdles they overcame to give us the life they did. We do our best to repay them, selflessly protecting the family *izzat* they cherish.

The guilt and shame used to ensure our compliance wrecks our mental health as we battle crippling anxieties over the safety of our ancestral heirloom. Kim argues this gut-wrenching shame impedes our self-confidence and hinders our success:

> "Shame, as it turns out, will more often than not sabotage rather than support a person's success—when success is defined more broadly as emotional, relational, and career thriving."

But, we can't seek any mental health support either.

A struggle with mental health would just be another crack in our family heirloom—a crack we wouldn't be able to sustain.

This guilt culture we have been brought up with has dimmed the light in so many eyes. Sagar, a Pakistani immigrant, remembers his cousin was reprimanded for posting videos on her YouTube channel. "My aunt told her she shouldn't be doing these things as a girl. That no one would marry her if she was embarrassing the family like that," Sagar told me. We're either forced to hide away our true identities and lives (and live with the fear and guilt of doing so) or sacrifice them (and live with the fear and guilt of doing so). We internalize the guilt over time, conditioned to shame and guilt ourselves.

Shame on us for not following our parents demands. Shame on us for not listening to our own needs and wants. At the end, we are left feeling like imposters in our skin.

Mardangi | Manhood

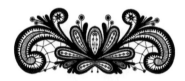

Dear Akaash,

Welcome to Manhood, baby brother. Today I finally get to teach you what it means to be a real man—a *mard*. Just as *Bapu* taught me and his *Bapu* taught him. I get to pass down traditions to you that we will get to pass down to our sons one day.

When I turned sixteen, *Bapu* wrote me a letter just like this one. He said to me:

Dear Jay,

As you become a man, you have to remember your manhood comes from your strength and your strength is all you really have. There's no room for weakness here.

*You must hold your head up high and do what you need
to do for your family. But, you can never ask for help.
Because a needy man is not a man at all.*

*You are a leader. A man always leads: the family, the
woman, the household. You get to make the decisions
and carry the family with you on your shoulders. There
is no room for error. As a man, you will be the provider of your family, the protector. And to protect, you
must be strong. To be a man, you need to look the part.
Maybe start hitting the gym more often. You should
work on being a little less scrawny.*

*The responsibility of providing for your family rests on
the man's shoulder. You are the provider. That is where
your mardangi comes from. Your family will depend
on you and only you. I won't lie; the burden is heavy,
but only you, alone, can carry it. There is no time to
waste with frivolous, girlish hobbies like that cooking
you seem so fond of. You are a man, you are the rock.
You must be unshakeable.*

I spent a lot of time making sure I lived my life as *Bapu* taught
me. He was so successful in his life, surely he had the correct
formula on how to be a real man? But, when I was twenty-one
years old, just figuring out what *mardangi* means, I learned
something *Bapu* never taught me. Though I wish he could
have taught me this, I don't think it's something he ever truly
understood himself.

My first girlfriend and I had just broken up. I thought Sai
was the love of my life. Losing her felt as though my world

was crashing down on me. I felt sad, hopeless, and downright miserable. I didn't know what to do. I was missing classes and didn't hang out with my friends much. My friend Andrew noticed I wasn't doing okay. I guess it was pretty obvious I was struggling. As we were walking back to our dorm after class one day, he asked me how I was coping with my breakup.

"I'm fine, bro. It's not a big deal. I just try not to think about it." I tried to brush him off and kept walking. I didn't want him to know how much I was really struggling. *Bapu* taught me that men couldn't ask for help; they had to hide their feelings. But, Andrew was persistent.

He stopped walking and stood in front of me. "I don't think ignoring your problem is going to make it go away. Plus, I think you are sadder about breaking up with Sai than you're letting on." He tried to look me in the eye, but I wouldn't let him and avoided making eye contact. "It's okay, bro. I just want to help you. I don't think keeping this all in will help you feel better."

"If I think about it, it makes me feel worse. I can't waste my time being sad. Men aren't supposed to talk about this stuff anyway, dude." *Did his father not give him the memo?*

Andrew shrugged. "That's what my older brother said too, man. But, I think that's bullshit. It's not fair that we have to just suck it up and keep going like nothing is wrong. If we keep it bottled up, we're going to burst one day. I'm gonna ask you again: are you sure you're feeling okay about this breakup? You look pretty depressed." He walked over to a nearby bench and sat down. He leaned forward and rested his forearms on his knees. Andrew looked at me, patiently waiting for me to join him. I gave in and sat down. In a moment of weakness, I let it all out.

"You're right." I sighed. "My breakup really sucks. I am actually really sad about losing Sai. I feel hopeless about it and I...I...I just don't know what to do." Suddenly, a tear rolled down my face. I was crying? In public? I felt embarrassed to be crying in front of Andrew, to be crying at all. I looked down toward the ground so no one walking by would see me like that.

At the same time, I felt like a burden had been lifted off my shoulders. Crying *actually* felt good. *Is this normal?* I explained to Andrew how distraught I really was and how lonely I felt. I didn't even realize I was feeling those emotions until I described them to him out loud. Andrew didn't even flinch or squirm at my tears. He listened to me and told me how he felt after his breakup the year before. He told me he had cried about it too and it was okay. Listening to him, I felt lighter, freer. I truly felt better. But it still felt weird to say these things out loud—it still felt like I was doing something wrong.

Twenty minutes into our intense conversation, a few of our other friends walked by. Marvin waved and said, "Hey, Andrew, Jay!" I quickly turned my head in the other direction so they wouldn't see me wipe my tears. "What's up, guys! You guys down to play to some ball?" Marvin and Aaron walked up to the bench we were sitting at.

I cleared my throat. "Hey, guys! Yeah, let's do it." I tried really hard to make my voice sound normal, but it was still a little shaky.

"Yo, Jay, what's up with your voice?" Aaron took a closer look at me. "Dude, were you crying or something?" He scoffed.

Marvin chimed in, "Nah, man, Jay is no pussy. I know he's not crying about that girl. That is some weak shit. Men don't cry. Right, Jay?" They both burst out laughing. *I knew I shouldn't have said anything.* I looked over at Andrew, hoping he wouldn't say anything about our conversation.

"C'mon, guys. Stop busting his balls. Jay doesn't cry. He's got nothing to cry about anyways," Andrew said, coming to my rescue. He knew I'd be humiliated if they knew, especially after their comments.

Bapu taught me men weren't supposed to show our emotions and I talked about my feelings anyways. I figured I deserved it when Marvin and Aaron made fun of me, made me feel like lesser of a man for crying. They were right. I had messed up.

But, were they? I spent these last five years trying to fix the mistake I thought I had made. I made sure to put on a strong front and bury my emotions, like a man is supposed to do. I never cried again after that day. I sucked it up and kept going, like a true *mard*. But somewhere, deep inside, I have desperately craved that feeling of freedom I felt when I shared my vulnerability with Andrew. I am exhausted from carrying this burden, holding everything in, and avoiding what I feel just to prove my manhood. There has to be a better way, right?

Even though it's what we were taught to believe, I realize now Marvin and Aaron were wrong. There's a better way. Twenty-one-year-old me was no less of a man because of the tears he shed. I won't lose my masculinity because I would rather spend my time baking than golfing. There's nothing weak or emasculating about me leaning on my friends for support, asking for help.

So as you learn to become your own man, Akaash, don't take *Bapu's* letter to me as the Holy Grail I thought it was. The truth is, there's no one way to be a man. Your *mardangi* comes from your courage to be yourself—to be human. So feel the sadness, and the grief. Let yourself cry and ask for help. These things don't take away from your masculinity. Rather, they will help you be a better, happier version of you.

Sincerely,
Jay, still learning (and unlearning) what it means to be a man

"Toxic masculinity" has been thrown around a lot in recent years. In 2019, Gillette released a commercial turning their original motto, "The best a man can get," on its head. They evolved their slogan into a call to action: "It's only by challenging ourselves to do more that we can get closer to our best." Portraying scenes of aggression, bullying, and catcalling, the commercial highlighted the evolution of the culture surrounding masculinity and the real harm it can do. Toxic masculinity refers specifically to the ideology that men must suppress their emotions, use violence for power and domination over others, and perpetuate misogynistic behavior. Boys are taught they have to be "tough" and can't show weakness (considered akin to femininity).

The expectation for boys and men to be "macho" or the "alpha male" leads to violent and aggressive risk-taking behaviors. Toxicity also comes from the lack of other options. We're told there is only one correct way to be a man—anything else isn't manly enough. This trepidation over destructive masculinity isn't just cultural, it's also a medical concern. The American Psychological Association (APA) outlined guidelines for working with boys and men who have been socialized with these "traditional masculinity ideologies" because they tend to be overrepresented in having social and emotional issues. According to the APA, "conforming to traditional masculinity ideology has been shown to limit males' psychological development, constrain their behavior, result in gender role strain and gender role conflict, and negatively influence mental health and physical health." The behaviors that boys are taught and exemplified through role models are unhealthy and put them at greater risk for long-term physical and emotional harm.

Social media now allows us a platform to discuss and begin to tackle the toxicity spread by such ideals, at least in Western culture. However, the same isn't happening in South Asian cultures, even though the harmful ideals of masculinity are far more pervasive and rigid. Young brown boys are habitually reminded—conditioned even—that they shouldn't "cry like girls" or "talk like girls." Boys are reprimanded for playing around with girls too much lest they become like them. I have personally heard aunties asking their sons why they're

sitting inside with the girls when they should be outside playing with the other boys.

Men are expected to be stoic, frigid, emotionless. If they don't
follow these expectations, their masculinity or sexuality is
immediately questioned. Sahil, a twenty-two-year-old Indian-American, questioned his own sexuality because he didn't
fit the typical masculine image expected of him. "You have
to be a strong, buff guy with no emotion, otherwise they
think you're gay," he said. If a man does express emotion,
he's corrected with "be a man," a reminder that he's doing
something wrong.

To preserve cultural gender norms, there's typically a physical separation between girls and boys from a young age and
through adulthood. This not only further exacerbates the
rigidity of the gender roles and expectations upon men, but
it also helps reinforce stereotypes of *mardangi*. Whether they
enjoy it or not, young men are expected to socialize only with
other men. Within these circles, they pick up the traits and
behaviors expected from men.

South Asian gender roles and the patriarchal structure prevent Desi men from accessing their emotions in the name of
tradition and culture. Along with these constraints, brown
men are immediately burdened with the task of being the
provider. They can neither shirk this responsibility nor share
it with a woman, otherwise their masculinity is doubted. Like
Jay mentions to his brother in the letter, men aren't allowed
to seek help without being considered weak. They must carry
the burden of providing for and protecting their families
without any space to process the scars that baggage leaves.

We see this at home and it's reinforced on screen. The trope of emotionally unavailable fathers in TV serials and movies is commonly found in our own homes. Bollywood never shies away from reminding its viewers that "*mard ko dard nahi hota* (real men don't feel pain)" (*Mard*, 1985). Whether it was Amrish Puri playing a distant, callous father in *Dilwale Dulhania Le Jayenge* in the nineties or Salman Khan using violence to solve his quarrels in every action movie since 2000, boys are constantly taught there is only one way to be a man. In her aptly titled opinion piece, "'Mere paas toxic masculinity hain'" (I have toxic masculinity),[4] Souraja Chakraborty explains the problematic nature of the "angry young man," often played by Amitabh Bachchan:

> "*He set to the youth a very problematic example of what a 'man' is. He is never vulnerable, and the only emotion a man is allowed to feel is anger and vengeance. A woman who is not interested in him will find herself in danger and eventually be at his mercy to be saved from her woes.*"

Bollywood's "angry young man" era (1960s–1990s), which gave us classics such as *Sholay* (1975), defined masculinity for our fathers (and us) by glamorizing charismatic heroes as they singlehandedly fought off groups of thugs to save their damsels in distress.

---

4 The title of this article is a play on a famous quote from a Bollywood movie, *Deewaar* (1975). The character proudly exclaims, "*Mere paas Maa hain*," meaning "I have a mother," when asked what valuable thing he has if not a car, bungalow, or "bank balance."

Our immigrant fathers, equipped with these inherited beliefs, are the toughest men we know. They always "held it together," kept their emotions and vulnerabilities in check to avoid being perceived as weak. The only emotions that men are allowed to display are anger and rage—so that's what they do. Unable to channel their emotions in other ways, immigrant fathers are forced to use aggression and anger as their only coping mechanism. Our fathers are angry because that's all they know to be. For them, their masculinity was only practiced through the power and control they could exert over others. What else should we expect from a generation that grew up watching hypermasculine "angry young men" celebrated on screen?

While the "angry young man" may have left the screen, Bollywood has found another way to promote hypermasculinity in the media. Images of extremely muscular men with glistening six-pack abs have now taken over. This time, *mardangi* is based on how many push-ups you can do and how low your body fat percentage is. This unrealistic image causes body dysmorphia, a psychological disorder involving an obsessive focus on a perceived flaw in appearance. In men, this obsession can lead to extreme and unhealthy behaviors such as drug abuse, over-exercising, and eating disorders. A report by National Eating Disorders Association discovered 25 percent of men in the US are affected by anorexia and bulimia. Often these eating disorders occur alongside depression- and anxiety-related symptoms.

These patriarchal norms, perpetuated by both men and women in our society, give boys a false sense of identity about their masculinity. Mothers, doting on their sons who can never do anything wrong, reinforce the idea that men and boys don't need to be held accountable for their actions. A young boy hitting a girl is just being naughty: boys will be boys. And when a man sexually assaults a woman, the response is the same. Throughout the years, "this common mentality has enabled and nourished some men, teaching them that consequences do not apply to them" (Manzanares, 2021). This is further cemented by strict patriarchal norms in Desi culture: women are subordinate to men. Be it a mother, daughter, sister, or wife, women aren't allowed to question men. So, who will?

Indian-American Krish recalled the double standards he witnessed at home while growing up: "As a son, you can commit murder and it would be fine. I was able to go wherever and do whatever, but my sister always had to stay with my mom." Similarly, thirty-two-year-old Gita told me that her much younger brother had a later curfew than her growing up. "I wasn't allowed to go many places or stay out with friends, but it was never a question for him," Gita recalled. These double standards solidify that women and men are expected to behave differently.

Playing within the bounds of masculinity and strict gender roles restricts men's abilities to form meaningful connections. They then suffer from loneliness and mental isolation. Ultimately, these behaviors cause mental health issues such as anxiety and depression because they are unable to cope with their trauma in a healthy way. Due to the stigma, Desi men aren't able to discuss their declining mental health, which makes their symptoms even worse.

While toxic masculinity is usually cited as harmful to women through perpetuating misogynistic behaviors, it is evident that it is equally as harmful to men themselves. Remedying toxic masculinity starts with freedom. Allowing men the freedom and space to express their vulnerabilities, their emotions, and their personalities will relieve them of the burdens they are forced to carry. Giving them the space to feel their weakness, reconcile with it, and learn healthy coping mechanisms for their struggles will prevent men from being trapped in the toxic cycle of masculinity. This all starts with men being willing, like Andrew was for Jay, to be vulnerable with their peers and to listen to one other. It starts with men encouraging other men to speak up about their issues and seek help when they need it.

Ammi ki Guriya | My Mother's Doll

Dear *Ammi*,

I wish I could say that I miss you. Perhaps a part of me does, but then I remind myself that there's no point. It's better to cut my losses and move on.

What do you see when you think of me, Ammi? I bet you see that ten-year-old girl with an embarrassing bowl cut, and a grin she thought would cover it up. You hear her words ringing in your ears, the words you always liked to hear: "Yes, *ammi.*" This ten-year-old girl is the doll you always wanted: *Ammi's guriya.* You dress her as you please, you play with her as you please, and you abandon her as you please. But only as *you* please. This is *your* doll, an extension of you—your flesh and blood. It's only fair that you get to decide the rules of all the games. After all, mother knows best.

She became your outlet, your escape. When things were good, *guriya* was your only priority, you poured every ounce of devotion you had into her. When things were bad, your doll was on the floor, hair torn out, discarded until things were good again. But in playing dress-up with your *guriya*, you forgot about the daughter she was. I strove to keep the skies clear as long as possible, because only then was your *guriya* showered with the love and adoration I so desperately craved.

"Being a woman is hard. You have only one chance. There's no room for mistakes. Don't ever let me down and don't let me look bad." That's what I hear ringing in my ears when I think of you. I see you, looking down at me with a trepidation in your eyes. As if any sudden movement I make will collapse the seemingly fragile reputation I have been destined to protect.

Your *guriya* was the apple of your eye, *Ammi*. She was your favorite toy to play with. Until she wasn't. The little girl who was showered with love and adoration became the young woman who no longer deserved it.

"You'll be happy when I die, then you can do whatever you want." Those words are etched into my brain along with the guilt that accompanied them. If losing you was the way to happiness, then I didn't want to be happy. I had decided long ago—well, *guriya* did—I wanted your love no matter how much it hurt. Anything was better than no mother at all, right? So I played the games you wanted me to play. The name of the game was success—nothing less was allowed. As a daughter, I already had more to prove to you and to the world than a son would. I had to prove I was more than the *guriya* you played with as you pleased, that I deserved the love you reserved for your princess doll. But even achieving the success you asked me to was never quite enough. The scars of my past failures were permanent. No matter what I did, it was only those scars you saw. Because my success was your success, but my failure was also your failure.

When I came home with a hole torn in my jeans, you never asked if I was okay. You got angry instead. When I came home with the highest grade in class, you didn't tell me you were proud. You told me not to let it get to my head. When I asked to see my friends, you didn't say yes. You told me that my family was enough.

But this family wasn't enough for me. Because I wasn't enough for them. *Ammi*, you always told me that those who had daughters were amongst the luckiest—*you* were amongst the luckiest. Why did I never feel lucky to *be* a daughter?

I don't know if you ever loved me. I think you only loved your *guriya*, never the girl inside her. But that wasn't enough for me. Zara needed love, she needed your trust.

The little *guriya* who could never live up to your ever-changing impulses went into the world eager to please everyone she met. She sought kernels of adoration wherever she went. They were the only form of love she knew, the only form of love she was allowed to have. She obsessively sought success after success, hoping this would be the one that made the difference.

Ammi, I tried my hardest not to let you down, but you always let me down. I don't want to be let down anymore. I don't need to wait for you to die to do whatever I want, to be happy. I don't need to wait for you to die to protect myself from you.

I choose to be happy now, even if that means leaving you and being your *guriya* behind. I protect myself today because I can. I protect myself today for the little *guriya* who had no one to protect her.

Goodbye,
Zara, the girl inside your *guriya*

P.S. I hated being your *guriya* and I'm glad I don't have to be anymore.

Sugar, spice, and everything nice? No—manipulation, control, and criticism. These are the ingredients used to create the perfect little *brown* daughter. The parenting techniques our families inherited normalized an abusive and codependent culture which has been cycling for generations. Starting from a young age, families socialize children, especially young girls, to follow strict gender roles by calling it culture. Parents and family members justify their strictness and demands as the status quo: "This is how *we* were raised." As I've mentioned before, there is an "us" (the immigrant family) and a "them" (the outside world). By using differences in culture, parents justify their controlling actions and toxic behavior as normal. Our parents' expectations are high. They expect us to achieve the greatness they came searching for when they left their homelands. They want their sacrifices to be worth it, and rightfully so. But the mechanisms used to ensure these expectations are met and far more toxic than the expectations themselves.

The parenting tools used to ensure expectations are met include criticism and humiliation. By constantly criticizing and comparing their children to others, mothers instill a sense of shame in their daughters. Anvi, a twenty-seven-year-old Sri Lankan-American, described her experience being compared to her cousins and friends: "You have such a nice figure. It would be so great if you could maintain it, unlike your cousin." Even if it was meant as a compliment, young girls internalize these comments, feeling ashamed for not fitting the desired image requested of them. Anvi described the immense pressure she felt being the topic of the aunties' conversations, especially after hearing comments when she gained weight during college: "Such a lovely girl, but now she has gained weight."

According to these aunties, Anvi's worth and value as a human were tied to her physical appearance. And with their comments, they instilled a sense of shame in her about her worth and desirability as a woman. Anvi recounted how she tried to do whatever she could to not be the topic of conversation, including skipping family events to distance herself from the critical eye of the aunties. Slowly, this desire for their daughters to fit a specific standard can turn into control. In an article about toxic parenting, Nivedita Jayakumar recalls her friends' mothers would put their daughters on liquid diets so they could "look good" for their dance performances or any other events where others might comment on their bodies.

The constant criticism from parents who are supposed to love us unconditionally leave many feeling disempowered and worthless. Growing up, we walked on eggshells, afraid of getting in trouble for the next wrong thing we did. In adulthood this presents itself as codependency. Licensed counselor Sharon Martin states these codependent traits can show up as "trying to fix or rescue others, acting like a martyr, perfectionism, overworking, wanting to feel in control, difficulty trusting, denial, guilt and shame, difficulty identifying and expressing your feelings, people-pleasing, anger, blaming, feeling unlovable, being self-critical, and not valuing yourself" (2017).

These traits are often the result of emotional abuse and constant criticism experienced during childhood. Because of these experiences, many of us have trouble in our adult friendships and romantic relationships. Divya, a twenty-eight-year-old Indian-American, recalled to me how she felt the "constant need to seek the validation [she] didn't get growing up, especially in romantic relationships." She mentioned feeling the need to overcompensate and "prove herself" to friends and boyfriends because of her insecurities. Similarly, Zara, from our story, consistently craved acceptance and trust from her mother and those around her. The unhealthy relationship with a toxic parent built on disapproval, fear, and manipulation left Zara, Divya, and many others questioning whether they were even deserving of love.

Our Desi parents often state these criticisms are for our "own good" or because they care. What they may perceive as their love language becomes the root of our insecurities and lack of self-esteem. What they hope motivates us and prevents us from being lazy ends up discouraging us and causing us to shut down. Down the line this constant criticism presents in feelings of misery, depression, or anxiety: "The anxiety is from the fear of not being good enough in the future. The depression from the discouragement of not having achieved enough in the past" (Kim, 2020).

Emotional blackmail is another toxic parenting norm that many South Asian kids have experienced. Often parents will use their parental care and nurturing as a bargaining chip. "We have done so much for you, is this how you will repay us?" It's not fair or healthy to use a scorecard in any relationship, but especially not in a parent-child relationship. By doing so, parents treat everything they've done as a debt their children must repay. In South Asian culture, though, this is often how parenting is viewed. Parents have several children as insurance policies to guarantee they'll be taken care of once they reach a certain age. This sends the wrong message to children; instead of: "I took care of you because I love you and I hope you will take care of me because you love me," the message sent is "I took care of you so you will take care of me. You must always do what I say to repay your debt, otherwise you are an ungrateful child."

In our story, Zara's mother told her: "You'll be happy when I die, then you can do whatever you want." This is another example of emotional blackmailing that utilizes parents' mortality as the bargaining chip. Sahaj Kohli, the founder

of Brown Girl Therapy, calls this "weaponized mortality."
Parents weaponizing their mortality to exert control teaches
their children they're "solely responsible for other people's
wellbeing, lives, and for maintaining the peace" (Kohli, 2020).
This tactic is so common it has become a trope in Bollywood
movies and South Asian TV serials. In Desi culture, parents
take on the responsibility of ensuring their children get married. It's not uncommon to see characters agree to marriage
to appease a grandparent or parent on their deathbed.[5] Yes,
our parents want to be a part of our happiness and see mile-
stones in our life—and so do we. But forcing us to "relieve
them of the burdens" of having to get their children married
rather than letting it happen organically is selfish.

Netflix's *Indian Matchmaking*, a show about an Indian
matchmaker matching Indian-American clients for marriage, included interviews of the clients' parents describing
their childhoods. In one episode, Aparna Shewakramani's
mom, Jotika, told her young daughters: "Please don't ever
let me down and don't let me look bad in our society, in
our community, nothing less than three degrees." Aparna's
mom convinced her children it would be *their* fault if their
mother was looked down upon in society. This emotional
blackmail plays up the prevailing idea that to express your
love for your family, you must sacrifice for them. In Desi
culture, putting your family ahead of yourself is the way
to show care. Later in the episode, Jotika excitedly recalled
how obedient her daughters were for repeating, "Yes, mama,"

---

5   This is in contrast to other cultures where parents also have a desire to see
    their children married but not the responsibility to ensure it. Setting up
    your daughter on a date is vastly different from compelling and forcing
    her to get married, no matter what it takes.

at her every command. Of course, there is nothing wrong with having children who listen to you (it's very desirable) or listening to your parents. What *is* wrong is parental care being bartered for obedience to commands that often dictate the paths of our lives.

Religion is another weapon parents often use to justify much of their toxic behavior. Our parents equate our religiosity with our worth. A good kid is the one who prays, otherwise they are labelled disobedient. Our relationship with our faiths is heavily scrutinized and even used as a measure of our success. Any pain or hardship you endure is assumed to be the consequence of faith deficiency. A mention of issues with mental health immediately questions how much faith a person has: "You are depressed because you don't pray." Children are guilted into practicing religion so their feelings won't be invalidated. We're told to pray the depression and anxiety away without diagnosing where the problem may be coming from. Religion used in this way often deters us from practicing it and believing in it at all. The more I was told to pray my depression away, the more I ran away from religion. I felt I had done something wrong and must deserve what I was feeling. What was the point of praying?

If we dare stand up against the blackmail and criticisms, it's immediately labelled as insolence. Telling our parents that our boundaries have been crossed or that we feel disrespected is of no use. We must either stay quiet and keep the peace or suffer the consequences of defiance. For some this means losing privileges, others lose their families. So then we're stuck, keeping the peace in order to keep our family. Boundaries violated and emotionally blackmailed, our mental health is threatened.

All of these comments and approaches to parenting constantly remind us that our parents' love comes with a long list of terms and conditions. The threat of causing shame to the family or being disowned looms over our heads constantly. But our parents' love shouldn't be conditional. We should be loved without having to earn it. We should be loved without fearing that tomorrow that love might be snatched away because we didn't follow certain expectations. We are worthy of love—real, unconditional love.

If the only love we're able to get from our parents is the toxic and manipulative kind, we may have to reconsider the value of that relationship. Is it serving us? Zara made the difficult decision to end her relationship with her mother. She chose emotional security over the constant rollercoaster of being loved and unloved by her mother. It's never easy to make this choice, especially for us South Asians. Our families and identities are a key part of who we are. But putting ourselves first is an important step in improving and rebuilding our mental health.

Pride

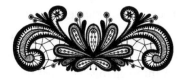

Dear sixteen-year-old Adam,

I know you've been feeling lost, confused, even ashamed for being who you are. You wish you could make it stop, make it not be true. I know how badly you want this to be a nightmare so you can wake up and stop feeling stuck, stop feeling so alone. You have knelt down in prayer time and time again, tears streaming down your face, begging, pleading for God to change you.

I can tell you now that those prayers will not be answered. You don't want them to be. There will be a day when you'll be glad they weren't answered. There will be a day when you'll get to be unabashedly who you are, *exactly* the way God intended. You won't have to hide who you are. Not from the world and especially not from yourself.

I'll be the first to tell you that your journey will be painful, arduous; there are still so many more tears to come. You'll be called names, judged before you even had a chance to be you. You'll be disappointed by the people you love, the ones you trusted.

When you see your family change the channel, make comments—repulsed by two men falling in love in a movie—you're afraid. It takes every ounce of your being not to flinch, not to show them how deeply their brazen comments wounded you. You think to yourself, *I don't want them to be repulsed by me. I want them to be proud of me.* This won't be the first time they hurt you like this, and this won't be the first time you'll want to change yourself for their sake.

When you feel like your community doesn't understand you (nor will they ever), you're not wrong. The whispers you hear at the mosque about others like you, they won't stop. Friends you grew up with will join in on the whispering too. The people who you prayed with on Fridays, standing shoulder to shoulder, your community, they will talk about how *those* people (people like you) are sinners, *kaafirs.* I know you try your hardest to hide yourself from them to ensure those whispers don't become *about* you.

I know listening to them, listening to the world deem your life an aberration, your feelings a sin, makes you feel disgusted. Not at them, but at yourself. I know you've tried your hardest to pray these feelings away, to beat them out of you, to cut them out of you. Your try to punish yourself, hoping this retribution will finally be enough for God to fix you. But he won't. **Because you don't need fixing.**

Do you remember when Mr. Henderson asked you in tenth grade what you wanted to be when you grew up? You made up some story about wanting to be an engineer, like your father. You figured that would suffice because you had gotten pretty good at convincing people with your fake stories. And it did. You didn't answer Mr. Henderson's questions truthfully. Far before then you had already decided you weren't even going to make it that far. You wouldn't be around long enough to have a career, so there was no point in picking one. There are so many things you didn't let yourself do and choose and feel because you had given yourself a deadline—an expiration date. You numbered your days and spent that time figuring out how to pull the trigger.

You're so afraid of believing in a future for yourself right now. Don't be. I am living proof your days are not numbered, not in the way you thought they were. I want you to dream big. Find the things that bring you joy. Feel joy. You're allowed to. You deserve to.

You're allowed to feel happiness and to have a life, even though so many people will tell you that you can't. It will hurt the most when those words come out of your mother's mouth. When she stops looking into your eyes and speaks only to your shadow. "*Log kya kahenge*? Where did I go wrong? Don't do this to us. You're going to go to hell."

You'll lose a family along the way. But I am here to tell you you'll gain a family along the way as well—one that chooses to love you. You'll build your own family, one in which people won't ask you to change or make you feel worthless: a family that will be proud of you no matter what. Together you'll be able to put back the pieces of yourself that you had broken off and that others had broken for you.

At the end of this journey, you'll find the home that your house could never be, a home I know you so desperately need right now. It'll be a place where you don't have to lower the pitch of your voice or hide who you love. One day you'll be able to speak with God again, this time not asking him to change you or erase you.

You'll still find it hard to forgive the people who hurt you. I am still struggling with that. But you don't have to forgive them, not until you are ready. Until then we can create a safe space for ourselves to heal, to learn, to grow. We can finally have a space to get to know ourselves. *What makes Adam happy? What does Adam like to do?* We'll be able to love ourselves because we **are** worthy of love. We'll make up for lost time and allow ourselves the chance to dream about a future—all the things we didn't think we would be around for.

There are so many wonderful things that await you, Adam, that await us. Amidst all the confusion, shame, and guilt, you made it this far. You should be filled with pride. Pride in who you are, who you will become, and even in the scars you have collected along your journey.

Sincerely,
a twenty-five-year-old PRIDEful Adam

South Asia has a long, complicated history with queerness. Prior to British colonization, the Indian subcontinent was no stranger to fluid sexuality and gender identity. The 1861 anti-sodomy law imposed by the British empire on the colonized greater Indian subcontinent profoundly altered the acceptance of fluid sexuality and gender identity in South Asia. For starters, the term "sexuality" was introduced as connected solely to gender and genital characteristics. Over time, "the Western concepts of heteronormativity and sexuality reinforced patriarchal structures and traditional gender roles already present in the society" (Bharat, 2015). The concepts brought over by the British laid the groundwork for discrimination and the social disenfranchisement of queer individuals in South Asia.

Today this translates to a deep-rooted stigma and internalized homophobia and transphobia in South Asian cultures, making coming out as a queer Desi that much more difficult. Even though both—the Western societies we immigrated to and the Eastern societies we left behind—have become much more accepting of the LGBTQ+ (lesbian, gay, bisexual, transgender, queer) community, immigrant parents continue to hold onto the antiquated mentalities they left with. Queer Desis often face backlash from their families and communities due to the stigma and shame still attached to the LGBTQ+ community. They could be disowned by their families during the process, or worse, forced to hide their identities and continue to live a double life. In other cases, those who have come out are met with emotional blackmail and violence.

The biggest fear for parents is that the Desi community finds out their child is queer. It's seen as sorrowful, something for others to pity. Parents are often more apprehensive about *log kya kahenge*, which makes coming out riskier and more traumatic. Even if some parents are willing to accept—or at least acknowledge—their identity, LGBTQ+ Desis have the added potential of losing their community, which is such an integral component in our collectivist culture. It's akin to an extended family, especially for immigrants, whose biological families are often back in South Asia. We grow up going to the church, temple, mosque, or mandir with our family-friends, usually dubbed cousins. Our communities are inextricably linked to our identities as South Asian immigrants. The possibility of being shunned or mistreated by the same community we consider to be our family makes coming out and living authentically a choice riddled with hurdles.

For those whose coming out is not welcomed by their family, the process is tougher. Pieces of identity are stripped away as if their culture, their religion, and their community is a privilege they no longer deserve. Religion is often the tool parents weaponize to guilt and shame their children, especially during the coming out process. Regardless of our own personal relationship with it, religion comprises a core piece of our South Asian experience. In fact, the communities we grow up in are usually based around our religious identities. Upon coming out, a Desi person's identity is deemed morally wrong: a sin. They're berated for following the "wrong path" and going against their religion—the same faith that taught them about love and acceptance.

> "When I first came out as a lesbian, my sister told me there was something terribly wrong me and my family tried to kill me, so I had to escape. They said I was possessed by Shaytan, the devil. I have lost my family, and have been treated as a kaafir by my siblings." (@ kamillahanwar)

In describing their experience coming out to their Muslim family, this twenty-five-year-old shows us how easily LGBTQ+ people are stripped of their religion and their family. Whether they wish to practice their religion or not, they're forbidden from identifying with it. This makes it difficult for those who do want to practice their faith, as they are left with no community with which to do so.

In coming out, many are also met with emotional blackmail by their parents. Some families force their kids to hide their identities for fear of what others will say. Some are forced to continue practicing religion in spaces that may not be welcoming. When she came out, Nazz, an Egyptian-American Muslim woman, "wore hijab for years against [her] will" (@ thequeermuslimproject). For many, navigating their identity is more about survival than thriving or acceptance. Like many others, Nazz continued wearing a hijab to appease her family and protect herself from the unwanted backlash or harassment she might face as a queer Muslim from a conservative family. Similarly, Adam, from our story, continued to attend religious prayers even when his peers made homophobic comments. For Adam and Nazz, the priority was to keep a low profile and not attract attention to their sexuality rather than embracing or accepting it. In cases like these, queer individuals don't get the opportunities to explore or truly come to terms with their sexuality because they're always focused on hiding.

Rejection by families and communities is a draining experience and, unfortunately, many Desi queer people are unable to find solace in queer spaces either. Most queer spaces are dominated by whites; South Asians are once again alienated from another community because of their identities (Hinkson, 2019). They often face fetishization in the queer community, creating yet another space where they can't be authentically who they are. A queer South Asian woman, Saranya, voices the disconnect she feels with the larger LGBTQ+ community in Toronto in an ethnographic study by Sonali Patel:

"When I was [in white queer spaces] in the past [...] you don't feel understood, lack of sense of belonging, and just like disconnected. It's a different experience as a [South Asian] queer person" (Patel, 2019).

It's impermissible for them to be queer in brown spaces and be brown in queer spaces—wherever they go, they cannot bring their whole self along. To exist and be accepted in either of these communities, they have to sacrifice a part of themselves. Another of Sonali's interviewees, Parvati, lamented that her identities were often invalidated: "'It's as if I must apologize for one [identity] to properly be the second.'" People ask patronizing questions such as "Are you just experimenting?" or "Are you fully gay?" denying the possibility of being South Asian and LGBTQ+ (Patel, 2019). This lack of representation in queer spaces can also make it difficult for LGBTQ+ kids to come out because they don't see others like them in the world. Not only does this makes them feel like they are doing something wrong by acknowledging their queer identity, but there is the possibility of not being able to find a community when they do come out.

Navigating an LGBTQ+ identity within the South Asian community is an emotionally grueling task. There is uncertainty and fear of abandonment at every turn. There's no doubt this journey negatively impacts the mental health of our queer brown friends. Feeling as if their existence is a blatant mistake and their feelings are invalid forces them to lose their sense of self-worth and self-esteem. When they are rejected by the community they thought was their own, they internalize that shame and judgment others project onto them. The emotional blackmail and grief queer Desis are met with from their communities and families are traumatic experiences, putting them at significant risk for PTSD (post-traumatic stress disorder). A Harvard study noted a much higher prevalence of PTSD in LGBTQ+ youth than their heterosexual peers (Roberts et al, 2012). While some may be able to find healthy coping mechanisms through supportive friends outside or even within their communities, not all are able to do so. LGBTQ+ individuals are twice as likely to abuse substances or self-harm as coping mechanisms, which makes taking care of their mental health more difficult.

As a South Asian community, we must do better to protect and support our queer friends and family. Not only must we work to create safe spaces for them within our communities, but we must also stand up for them when they can't stand up for themselves. As we lift up the rest of our community, we can't leave our LGBTQ+ kids behind.

PART 3:

MOVING FORWARD

Awareness and acknowledgment that there's a problem is the first step. Next, we have to do something about it. While we learn about and reconcile the toxic and harmful parts of our society, we have to simultaneously prioritize protecting our mental health alongside that. It's also necessary to do so as we heal from the collective traumas that we, as a generation, have faced.

Nurturing our wellbeing helps us combat and proactively prevent poor mental health and physical illness. When we're mentally healthy, we're not just happier, but we're also better equipped to face the difficult life events that may come our way. Being mentally healthy doesn't mean you won't go through bad times, but it does mean you'll be able to bounce back from adversities that are a part of the rollercoaster of life.

We should all find ways to better our mental health so we can focus on thriving in our lives and not just surviving them.

Proactively working on your mental health will allow you to be resilient in the face of difficult experiences, maintaining a positive outlook even during uncertain times. Of the many ways to take control of your mental health, I discuss practicing self-care, building boundaries, seeking therapy, and having difficult conversations about mental health with our families. These strategies will not only help you better cope with any mental health struggles, but they will also help break the stigma surrounding mental health in our Desi communities.

Self-Care

#SelfCare #Mindfulness #Motivation
#Wellness

Self-care is about much more than just a slew of trending hashtags. As of late, it has become a buzzword, an Instagram aesthetic. It has become more about *looking* like you are taking care of yourself than *actually* taking care of yourself. That post-yoga selfie or self-care mantra on your feed is great to look at, but it's also a reminder of how crucial it is to properly take care of yourself. The term "self-care" really describes any action you *deliberately* take to prioritize and care for your mental, physical, and emotional wellbeing, especially during stressful times. Stress is a normal part of life. But when it goes unmanaged, it can make matters worse and negatively impact your mental health. Staying ahead of the curve and keeping up with day-to-day self-care habits can help us better mitigate stress and keep our mental health in check. You don't have to be officially diagnosed with a mental illness (i.e., depression, anxiety disorders, post-traumatic stress disorder) to make self-care a priority, though it's especially important for people who are. At the end of the day, self-care is really about maintaining a healthy life. And that can mean different things for different people.

Self-care not only looks different from person to person, but it also looks different for you at different times. So the bath bombs, candles, and wine that you see on #SelfCareSunday may work for your friends, but they don't have to work for you. When you are identifying your needs, they may look different every time you check in with yourself. Sometimes you may need that relaxing bubble bath, and other times you may need a nice long nap. Not all self-care activities will have that perfect Instagram aesthetic—that's okay. You are taking care of yourself for *you,* not your followers.

Sometimes you might even have to do something you don't really feel like doing in the moment (like my personal hell: running). What helps me in those moments is to remind myself I am doing this to help my future self feel better. It feels like less of a drag when I can point at what I will get out of it in the future. It won't always be easy, especially when you need it the most. The self-reflection required to prioritize your own care will ask you to be honest with yourself about your current state—the good, the bad, and definitely the ugly. It might require letting go of toxic habits or relationships that might be in your way. Getting started is usually the hardest part. The rest is about building a routine within your life.

Self-care is not just for when you are feeling in a funk or are actively dealing with mental illnesses; it's something that should be integrated within your lifestyle. It's important to make self-care a part of your routine, be that daily, weekly, or monthly, to protect and preserve your mental health. When these practices are integrated into your lifestyle, they will be much easier to execute when your mental health may not be at its best. It is much more difficult to start a new habit when you are already feeling down or depressed than going about a preestablished routine you are familiar with. It is in those moments that self-care matters the most. Creating a self-care routine is your best defense to be prepared for managing the normal stresses of life and cycles of struggles with mental health. It is a habit that must be maintained, adjusted, and readjusted as your life and your needs change.

Additionally, taking care of yourself on a recurring basis will help you be the best version of yourself and allow you to accomplish the goals you have set out for yourself. Feeling fulfilled mentally, physically, and emotionally will enable you dedicate yourself to accomplish the personal, professional, and social goals and responsibilities you espouse. As it is commonly said, "You cannot pour from an empty cup." If you fail to take care of yourself, you will never be able to do the same for others around you. This will only burn you out faster, and harder. Pouring from your cup into others' goes beyond simply taking care of your friends and loved ones. If you are not in the right headspace, it will be impossible to accomplish the necessary tasks for your job, school, or other commitments. When the burden of your neglected tasks starts to grow, your mental health will be negatively affected. Cue a downward spiral. You are burnt out. And now, you will not be able to give your energy to anything: your work, school, family, or friends.

When thinking about self-care, the key is to make your actions intentional. Taking care of yourself requires paying attention to your unique needs and creating a plan to address those needs. While they are important, your needs are not limited to the biological or physiological necessities we first think of when it comes to self-care, like hydration or eating a healthy diet. When considering your needs, look holistically at your mind, body, spirit, and emotional self.

You hear and feel your stomach growl. You immediately know you have a need: hunger. But not all needs will be as easy to identify as physical ones. In fact, sometimes it will be impossible to pinpoint exactly what your mind or body needs in the moment. It is important to think about which of your needs are currently unmet and what you can do to meet those needs in the moment. As you do this, ask yourself these questions:

- What are my current coping strategies? Do they help me cope with my stress in a positive way or do they make me feel more stressed?
- What do I value in my life every week?[6]
- What do I find missing in my life every week?
- What areas in my life do I most often neglect? How does that make me feel?

---

6 Breaking this down on a weekly basis will help you stay narrowly focused on solutions that can be implemented and produce results faster. It is also valuable to zoom out and think about this on a monthly or even yearly basis as a secondary step.

- What self-care practices am I already utilizing? Are they working for me? How can I add, subtract, or augment them?
- What obstacles are currently preventing me from practicing self-care habits?
- How can I remove these obstacles or work around them?

Asking these questions will help you take stock of your current self-practices as well as identify what may be lacking in your routine. A better awareness of your needs comes not only from self-reflection, but also by trying various self-care techniques to determine what fits best in your lifestyle. As you incorporate time to think intentionally about your needs, you will become better and faster at identifying them. It might be as simple as recognizing your triggers. If after this self-reflection you have come to the conclusion you are not someone who needs self-care, you are wrong! Your version of self-care might not like what you expect it to. But, <u>everyone needs to take care of themselves: physically, mentally, and emotionally.</u> It's a package deal.

At the end of the day, self-care is your responsibility. No one can come and do it for you (I would love to outsource my 5K runs sometimes). You may find a partner (a friend, mentor, sibling, parent) to practice some habits or strategies with you, but the onus to take care of *your*self is on **you**. It is your responsibility to yourself, to those who depend on you, and to those you care about. And if you don't carry out this responsibility, there are going to be some consequences for your mental, physical, and emotional wellbeing. The symptoms of neglecting your self-care will show up physically, mentally, as well as emotionally. The physical evidence will be obvious: exhaustion, body aches, muscle fatigue. You might notice a rapid change in your weight and the health of your hair and skin. Mentally, you may feel a "brain fog," characterized by a lack of mental clarity, poor concentration, and inability to focus. You may also feel the onset of symptoms such as low self-esteem, apathy, and difficulty in relationships. Author of *The Self-Love Workbook* Dr. Shainna Ali reminds us neglecting self-care can have serious consequences to our mental and physical health (Ali, 2019). If disregarded, these emotional symptoms can develop into longer-lasting mental health issues such as depression and anxiety.

SELF-CARE FOR SOUTH ASIANS

As I've mentioned, in South Asian culture self-sacrifice is celebrated, and self-care is the antithesis of that. From a young age, we see our parents portray this strong work ethic: they "work long hours, eat on the go, neglect rest, and rarely take a vacation" (Jacob, 2018). We learn to associate hard work and success with not taking a break. In *Brown Girl Magazine*, Steven Jacob describes how this learned "no-days-off mentality" promoted unhealthy competitive behaviors amongst his friend group from a young age:

> *"As friends tend to do, we've often looked for ways to turn this into a game, finding ways to compete in who can work harder. The commonly accepted belief is if you need rest, your hustle is invalid—and you don't have the mindset necessary for success. Needless to say, that mentality is not only ridiculous, but also harmful to our wellbeing" (Jacob, 2018).*

This ideology is not only harmful to us, but also to those who look up to us and inherit these detrimental habits. We are human and we need to take care of ourselves, take breaks, and cope with the stresses of life. If we do not find ways to do this intentionally, our brains still find a way. Often, the brain's last-ditch effort for release is not the healthiest coping mechanism and ends up creating more harm than good. These negative coping strategies might include excessive substance abuse (drugs and/or alcohol), over/undereating, self-isolation, or extreme aggression and anger toward those around you. While some of these outlets may provide a temporary release, they are not long-term solutions to the stressors of life. Proactively practicing self-care will allow you to incorporate positive and healthy coping strategies instead of unhealthy ones.

The most important thing to remember about self-care is it is, by no means, a selfish act. <u>I repeat: self-care is not selfish!</u> There is no act more self*less* than taking care of ourselves for the sole purpose of showing up whole for others. We may have been told growing up that taking a break is frivolous, a waste of time or money. But that is simply not the case. Taking care of yourself is not showing *nakhre*. You do not always have to "tough it out." Taking a break is not a weakness; it is your strength. Taking time for your mental, physical, and emotional wellbeing will help you be more capable for others. While our parents' generation, especially our mothers, were derided for taking care of themselves, we can break the cycle of this generational trauma by intentionally embracing self-care. When we show up for ourselves—authentically and intentionally—we are not only building stronger, more resilient versions of ourselves, but we are also setting an example for the next generation. Whether implicitly or not, we learn from our elders. Just as Steven Jacob learned to turn his hustle into a harmful competition, we have all inherited this hesitancy to take care of ourselves. By replacing this hurtful habit with a few restorative practices, we can introduce healthy self-care into our lives and pass it down to the next generation.

For those living in a Desi household, it may be difficult to practice self-care around parents or at home. It is important to think about how you can work around this obstacle and still take care of yourself. It may be the approach you thought of first may not be the most feasible to practice at home. Really think of alternative approaches to get what you need to take care of yourself. This could include involving your family in some of your self-care practices. Our parents don't have the best track record of taking care of themselves. Use this as an opportunity to help them incorporate some practices into their life as well.

Sometimes the self-care you need will require time away from your family. Use self-care practices to find pockets of time for yourself. The physical act of being away from home will make you feel rejuvenated and help you be more purposeful with the time you do get to spend with your family. The best way to do this in a household that is restrictive is signing up for an activity that requires you be out of the house. If that is hard to do, get creative with carving out time alone. Offer to pick up the groceries or run errands by yourself. Take your time, stop for a coffee on the way, and use your driving time as a pocket of peace. Driving has long been a go-to when I needed to clear my head. There is a sort of therapeutic quality to it that lets you take a break from the world while still actively cruising through it.

STRATEGIES FOR SELF-CARE

In the remainder of this chapter, I lay out some strategies for self-care that are recommended by experts, by friends, by interviewees, and by me. As you find ways to introduce self-care into your lifestyle, ask yourself the questions listed in the beginning of this chapter. After some reflection, pick a few strategies from below that will fit into your lifestyle, and be something you *actually* see yourself practicing. Remember self-care is **not** one-size-fits-all!

CARE FOR YOUR BODY:

- **Be active:** This will look different for everyone, but regular exercise helps improve mood and keeps your body healthy. You don't need a gym membership or any pricey equipment. Take a walk, go on a jog, ride a bike, practice yoga, grab a jump rope. Getting your body moving, in whatever way you can, even helps improve your sleep quality. If this is new for you, start out by incorporating physical activity once or twice a week into your routine. As your body gets used to this new habit, you can slowly increase the intensity and timespan of your activity.
- **Proper nutrition:** Eating healthy, balanced meals is key to ensuring your body is getting all the vital vitamins and minerals necessary for proper organ functions. Start by incorporating fruits and vegetables if they are not already a part of your diet. Make

sure you are eating enough calories and not skipping meals.

- **Drink water:** Hydration is key.
- **Get enough sleep:** Health professionals recommend seven to eight hours per night. If you have trouble accomplishing that, try limiting caffeine later in the day and avoiding "screen time" right before bed.
- **Limit reliance on alcohol, tobacco, or drugs:** Know and understand your limits. Excessive use of substances can contribute to poor mental health and exacerbate other symptoms of self-neglect.

CARE FOR YOUR MIND:

- **Meditation:** There are tons of free guided meditation videos that you can find online to follow along with. For those who are new to meditation, start with shorter meditations and work your way up. All you need is a quiet space and something to play your meditation audio on. Try this before bed or when you wake up.
- **Breathwork:** If meditation is not something you're able to do, try breathwork. Breathwork intentionally changes and manipulates the breath for an extended period of time. You can also find guided breathwork videos online to help you practice.
- **Journaling:** It may seem like a daunting task, but just pick up a pen and paper or open up a blank document and write out your thoughts. Culturally, we're conditioned to actively avoid our feelings. Use journaling as your time to sit with and confront the feelings you have learned to push aside. If you have

trouble starting, find some journal prompts online to spark some ideas. There is no word count or page limit here, just you and paper.

- **Unplug from social media:** Yes, social media is a great way to keep in touch with family and friends. But, too much "doom-scrolling" can leave you feeling anxious and exhausted. It is important to be intentional about your social media usage so the experience remains an enjoyable one. Unfollow (or mute) people who stress you out. Follow accounts and pages that make you feel happy and inspired. Limit how much time you spend on social media in a day. You can do this by setting reminders on your phone or structuring times when you check your social media. For example, read the news only when you're drinking your morning coffee or on your lunch break. If it gets to be too much, try deleting your apps for a few days or weeks to "cleanse" from overconsumption.

- **Read for pleasure:** Reading for pleasure is not the same as the reading you have to do for school or work. It may be about the same topics, if those topics will help you recharge. Reading is a way to learn something or experience something new. It is an easy way to unplug from screens that still leaves you feeling inspired. This practice became really hard for me during grad school when I had mountains of readings to do for my classes. But, I found every time I did get a chance to read something not school-related, it left me feeling calmer. If reading physical books doesn't work for you, try an audiobook.

- **Spirituality:** Many of us have complex relationships with our spirituality because of the overbearing cultural emphasis on religion. Spirituality as self-care can be what you want it to be. For some, that may look like spending extra time on prayers or reading religious texts. For others, you may find different methods express your spirituality. Find the practices that give you a sense of peace and calm—not the ones you feel obligated to do.

CARE FOR YOUR SOUL:
- **Build and nurture your relationships:** Find time to make meaningful connection with friends. Sometimes in South Asian households, friendships are not given priority; some of us only get to see our friends at school. If that is the case, use texting, social media (even e-mail if you are in a situation where your social media and texts are being monitored), and other ways to communicate and nurture your relationships with friends. It may not be ideal, but you don't have to feel guilty about hiding your friendships. Spending time with friends is important for our mental health and personal growth.
- **Reevaluate toxic friendships:** As important as friends are, they heavily influence us in ways we may not even realize. If your network is not as supportive as you need and is draining you, rethink it. Surround yourself with people who you are comfortable being yourself around!
- **Get creative:** Arts and crafts are a great way to destress and find a change of pace. Creativity can mean whatever resonates with you: music, dancing,

cooking, art. You don't have to be good at it. It just has to bring you joy.

- **Find a new hobby:** As I've discussed elsewhere, hobbies aren't always prioritized in some Desi households. Think about hobbies that intrigued you growing up. If there are things you didn't get a chance to engage with, try them out now.
- **Volunteer:** Find a cause you are passionate about and volunteer your time for them. You can use this time to work on a skill you have been developing or simply to make new friends. This is a great option for those who may have more restrictive family boundaries. Volunteering can be a way for you to get acquainted with a new environment and gain some space from your household.

CARE FOR YOUR SELF:

- **Set up boundaries:** Boundaries can be a complicated concept for Desi people. It's not something we are used to doing and can be very difficult at first. But boundaries are necessary to protect yourself and your mental health. In the next few chapters, I'll discuss more about how to set boundaries and why they are necessary.
- **Seek help when you need it:** Regularly practicing some of the above strategies will help you take care of yourself most of the time. But sometimes, you will need to lean on others to help you through a tough time. You may choose to lean on friends or family for extra support. If a larger crisis arises in your life or you notice your self-care plan is not working for

you, you might need to reach out to a professional. Yes, therapy. Because of the stigma associated with mental health, therapy is looked down upon and misunderstood. In the next chapter, I'll discuss how therapy can be a helpful resource for you.

These lists above are not exhaustive. Use them as jumping-off points to incorporate intentional self-care in your life. This may be an unfamiliar path for some of you. Start small. Self-care isn't going to fix everything. As Dr. Ali said, "[It] isn't a magic pill. There is not a single form of self-care that will have lasting effects with a sole effort" (Ali, 2019). This is something that will be (and should be) ongoing throughout your life. You're not doing this to check boxes. It should be a practice that is sustainable, one that requires active attention to all the parts of you.

Therapy

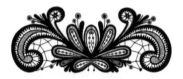

As Desis, we are conditioned to believe therapy is for the weak, for the "crazy" people, or for rich folk who have too much time and money on their hands. Learning more about what therapy is all about isn't even seen as an option. Therapy becomes, and stays, an elusive and foreign concept: something we don't talk about or attempt.

Seeking therapy is not an easy thing for most people. It's definitely not the first thing on the self-care checklist, and due to logistical difficulties (finding a therapist, making an appointment, etc.), it's also not the most straightforward process. While the millennial generation has significantly helped to normalize therapy and reduce the stigma associated with it, those extra hurdles are ever-present for South Asians, millennial or not. Through the use of social media, therapists and mental health advocates have been able to demystify therapy for the masses. But still, we are not really sure how therapy can be a tool for *us* to use. We may be aware of therapy as an option, but old habits die hard. We revert back to what we heard growing up: *therapy is not for brown people.*

WHAT CAN THERAPY DO FOR YOU?

According to the American Psychological Association, therapy is a treatment designed to relieve emotional stress and find solutions to problems in a collaborative environment. Therapists provide an objective, neutral, and nonjudgmental perspective to help people develop more effective problem-solving and coping skills. There are several types of therapy, but the most common is individual talk therapy (psychotherapy): you and the therapist talk openly in a confidential space to work through your struggles.

Therapy is extremely beneficial not only to those who are managing a chronic mental illness, but also to anyone who wants to learn how to better manage feeling overwhelmed or stressed. Therapy provides an outlet, a place to learn healthy coping mechanisms, all with the help of a professional. By talking through a situation with a therapist (sometimes called counselors), you gain a "third-party" perspective that you may not have seen before. They can serve as a sounding board for you when you are unsure how to handle a situation. Even just having the space to talk about a problem out loud and explain it to another person is a helpful benefit of therapy. So, if we just have to talk to someone, why can't we just talk with our friends? Or our parents (as they have suggested many times)? Why do we have to tell our business to someone else? It's a private, family matter, I don't want others to know about this and judge me.

Therapy isn't just a place to chat and gossip about family drama with another person, nor is it a place where you have to worry about confidentiality. Working with mental health professionals is beneficial because the coping strategies, tips, advice, and other techniques you learn and discuss are evidence-based and come from their clinical expertise. A therapist goes through extensive training, supervision, and licensure before you get to sit in that chair in front of them: "In most cases, becoming a therapist will take at least around seven to fifteen years following graduation from high school. Most therapists need a bachelor's degree, and then a master's degree, or a doctoral degree. Formal education is followed by supervised clinical hours of direct experience before one can become licensed as a therapist. This means that if one already has a bachelor's degree, it is a matter of four to ten years before they can be licensed as a therapist" (Selva, 2021).

Therapists are also bound by strict doctor-patient confidentiality laws that protect your privacy. The only time a therapist may have to disclose private information without your consent is if they are doing so to protect you or others from harm. For example, if a client discusses plans to attempt suicide, to harm another person, or if they report domestic abuse or neglect of a minor. These serious exceptions are in place to protect you and those around you. This plays out slightly differently if you are under eighteen. Often parents are involved when minors receive therapy services. According to the APA, "different states have different ages at which young people can seek mental health services without informing parents"

(2021). Be sure to check online for your state's 'age of consent law' on a government website.

There are two broad buckets of mental health professionals that offer psychotherapy services: psychiatrists and therapists. A psychiatrist holds a medical degree and focuses on treating and diagnosing mental illness. As doctors, psychiatrists are able to prescribe medication to their patients, but don't necessarily provide consistent talk therapy services. On the other hand, therapists are mental health professionals who only provide psychotherapy. Therapists cannot prescribe medication. When deciding which type of mental health provider to go to, the online counseling platform BetterHelp recommends thinking about your preferred treatment path, which can include medication, therapy, or a combination of the two. BetterHelp recommends consulting "with a psychiatrist or your primary care doctor if you want to consider medication. If you plan to incorporate a type of therapy, talking with a therapist is a good first step" (Thomas, 2021).

WHAT HAPPENS DURING THERAPY?

What comes to mind when you image a therapy session? You lie down on a couch in a softly lit office and talk while a therapist listens to you and takes notes, occasionally asking "How do you feel about that" or "Tell me more." Hollywood may have painted this picture about therapy sessions but, like most things Hollywood portrays, that's not exactly how it goes down. There are couches, and you *can* lie down if you want to, but a therapy session is more than just you monologuing out loud while someone takes notes. Sessions with a therapist are meant to be much more interactive than that. The first few sessions with a therapist will consist of you talking more than the therapist. But that is so the counselor can get to know you and your background. As they learn more about you and build a rapport, the therapist will not only ask you questions, but also provide suggestions, advice, and strategies to help reframe your thoughts.

Going into your first therapy session might feel overwhelming. *What am I supposed to talk about? Where do I start? Do I just tell them my whole life story?* There can be a lot of uncertainties when you start. It's important to remember therapy is a process. You're not going to go in for one session and suddenly feel better or have a new outlook on life. You might feel better after a certain therapy session, but that won't be the case every time, and that's okay. You may have an *Ah-hah!* moment during a session or you could leave feeling more confused than when you came in. That is all a part of the process. As overwhelming as it may seem, you just have to start by bringing up one issue—probably the one that finally convinced you to start therapy in the first place. It can be as general as "I don't feel like myself lately" or something more specific: "I'm struggling to deal with a loss in my life." As you start discussing your thoughts and feelings with your therapist, other issues and concerns will gradually come out. You don't have to lay it all out in one go. Our thoughts, actions, and feelings are often more connected than we think. As you bring them up to your counselor, they will start to recognize and identify connections you might not have realized are there.

Working with a therapist takes time and is an incremental process. There is also no linear trajectory. Your life is still going on around you and, while you might be working on addressing long-term issues, some short-term issues might get in the way and need to be addressed first. Studies have shown change can often be discontinuous and nonlinear (Hayes et al, 2007). There will be bumps along the way, times when change is really fast and when it is really slow. As you go through the emotional processing and meaning-making, you will likely disrupt some old patterns, learn to think differently, and create new habits. In my own experience there were times when I left a session elated because I finally understood something about myself and other times when I left upset because I realized I needed to change something. Going through this process will not always be easy, but it will definitely be worth it in the end. In describing his year and a half of therapy, Steven Jacob from *Brown Girl Magazine* mentioned:

> *"I can confidently say I'm a different person today. I've learned to be more compassionate and patient with myself, two things I struggled with in the earlier parts of my life. I have more fulfillment in my life and enjoy more meaningful relationships with the people around me. But the epiphanies and insights didn't come overnight"* (Jacob, 2018).

Therapy is not a one-way interaction—it's a conversation between you and the therapist. They talk to you as much as you talk to them. In fact, that's the benefit of having a therapist. As a third-party and neutral person in your life, your counselor will be able to zoom out and see a part of the bigger picture that you might be missing. They will provide a new perspective that you may not have considered. Because therapists see different clients daily, they'll even be able to pull suggestions from their work with another client. When we are bogged down by emotions in the middle of a situation, we tend to judge ourselves harshly. Working with a therapist will give you the space to be vulnerable about your true thoughts and feelings. There have been times when I was embarrassed to tell my therapist what I truly thought. I even told her how ashamed I was for thinking that way and how hypocritical I felt. But with the honesty and vulnerability, we were able to figure out how to change that narrative and how I could be more understanding and forgiving of my own shortcomings.

Though we wish it were true, there is no magic book with all the answers, and therapists can't wave a wand to make things all better. There is often not even a single answer or solution to the issues we may have. The goal of therapy is to work with a professional and learn the tools necessary to best respond to situations in your life. You should aim to understand why you feel the way you do and how your past experiences affect your actions and reactions. Your therapist will definitely not tell you what to do. They will instead advise you on what the healthy way to approach your situation may be. They will walk through your thoughts on how to respond or deal with something. At the end of the day, the decision is up to you on how you react. Whether you did the "right" or the "wrong" thing (there is often not really a right or wrong thing, but we are conditioned to compartmentalize as such), your therapist will be there to process it with you. They will not judge you for doing x instead of y. Instead, they will work through the situation with you, provide insight to your decision, and figure out a plan to move forward.

Most therapists acknowledge that much of the "therapy" actually happens outside of therapy. A single one-hour session per week or month is not enough to bring about the change or improvement you want. You should be prepared for some homework. Some therapists will actually give you homework at the end of a session. This can include spending time thinking or journaling about what you discussed, making observations about your thoughts and feelings as situations develop, or practicing the strategies they recommended. Only by implementing what you are learning in therapy will you begin to see its effects. There may be some trial and error on the coping strategies they suggested, but you won't know until you try them out. Just as with school, work, or any skill, you get out of it what you put into it. Showing up to therapy and being vulnerable and open during your session is only a part of the process, albeit a key part.

WHY DESIS (AND EVERYONE ELSE) NEED THERAPY

As a big proponent of therapy, I believe every adult should be required to seek consistent therapy for one year. It should be a required course in twelfth grade or the first year of college or university. There are innumerable benefits to therapy that go beyond addressing serious mental health concerns. For Desis, specifically, therapy provides a safe space to understand our mental health journey—a concept that is usually foreign to most of us. There are actually no words in our languages (and thus our frame of mind) to describe the scars left by generational trauma from the immigrant burden (see Part Two). So, we often do not know this trauma even exists. Not all of us will have this trauma, but our immigrant experience significantly increases the likelihood that we do.

Working with a therapist can teach you how to set better boundaries for yourself and others around you. Boundaries are either nonexistent, not enforced, or violated in collectivist cultures. We don't grow up seeing how crucial boundaries are nor examples of how to set them. A therapist can walk us through what boundaries may look like for us in the context of our culture. In the next chapter, I detail more about the importance of setting boundaries.

Seeking therapy can help us work through the identity conflicts, guilt, shame, and emotional burdens we have carried as first-generation children of immigrants. As a confidential space, we can use therapy to unpack the double lives we often have to live, without fear of judgment or backlash.

We can also use therapy to figure out how to set boundaries or have the difficult conversation about mental health with our families. The next chapters go into more detail about how to approach those conversations. A therapist is an excellent confidant to practice boundary-setting and discussing mental health with your family.

Lastly, the more of us who seek therapy, the more we can normalize it as a practice in our community. By actively taking care of our mental health in this way, we can work to break the stigma that therapy is for "crazy" people. It's not. Therapy is for everyone. We can all benefit from talking things through with a professional. I have recently gotten into the habit of bringing things my therapist taught me into conversation with my parents. At first, they would squirm a little, get uncomfortable with me acknowledging I go to therapy. After doing this a couple times, I noticed they started to squirm less and listen more intently. I even received some follow-up questions about what I was learning through therapy. By opening up like this, I showed my parents how I was actively working to take care of my mental health and how important it was to me. If we, as a generation, open up about our mental health, we can help normalize utilizing therapy or medication as options to take care of ourselves.

KNOW BEFORE YOU GO

Mouth agape, she scoffed. "Your mom should not be forcing you to get married! That is wrong of her." My therapist assumed my mother's incessant questioning about marriage and finding a boy were akin to forcing me to get married. I explained I wasn't being forced into anything and marriage has a different significance in the South Asian culture. I had actually come to the session to discuss how to cope with moving to a new city. Twenty minutes later, I was still defending my Pakistani heritage as not backward to my white therapist.

Lack of cultural competency is a major issue in mental health spaces—one that is especially relevant to us as South Asians seeking therapy services. In fact, Asian Americans underutilize or abandon mental health services at higher rates due to lack of cultural competency (Kim-Goh et al, 2015). When clients don't feel understood or feel they have to spend more time explaining or defending their culture than discussing the issue they were concerned with, like I did, therapy might end up doing more harm than good. A culturally competent provider is both aware of their biases and preconceived notions, and also actively "attempts to understand the worldview of his or her culturally different client." They work with their client to ensure they are "actively developing and practicing appropriate, relevant, and sensitive intervention strategies and skills" (Sue and Sue, 2008).

As I have discussed throughout Part Two, many of our mental health struggles as children of South Asian immigrants are rooted in cultural practices, the emotional distress associated with managing and forming identities, and the intergenerational traumas and burdens passed down to us. It's difficult to bring and unpack these experiences in therapy because most of the time we don't even realize they are there. We have to rely on our therapists to decipher the line between cultural quirks and actual cultural trauma.

Working with a therapist who is culturally competent is an essential first step.

Such a therapist will understand the cultural limitations we may be under and work with us to develop a strategy that works to reduce the friction caused by our culture rather than exacerbate it. A British-South Asian, Coco Khan, described how her experience turned her off from therapy for years. When her therapist advised her to completely cut off certain family members, she explained how the collectivist South Asian family structure made that difficult:

> *"Each week, she would ask me if I had yet severed the ties. I felt ashamed when I said I hadn't, as though I was a disappointment to her. It made our sessions tense and unproductive."*

As was mine, many of our first experiences with therapy occur during our college years with student health services. Most colleges and universities provide some sort of free short-term mental health services to students. Sometimes they become the first *and* last attempt at seeking therapy. During my time, students were allotted twelve free sessions per school year. After that, you were on your own, with a referral to external mental health services in hand. However, these services are generally more available on paper than they are in reality. While the prevalence of mental health struggles and issues amongst college students has dramatically increased in the past ten years, the supply of supportive services is not on par. In some cases, wait times can be as long as three weeks, which may not seem like much, but is nearly half an academic quarter (a lot can happen in half a quarter) (Thielking, 2017). Waiting large amounts of time between sessions or even for a single session reduces the efficacy of therapy, as neither a rapport nor a proper treatment plan can be devised when students are only seen during crisis mode. The lack of consistency in sessions and possibly even the therapist can hinder progress. It's only when things are at the point of safety and security risks that students are able to jump the line and be seen—that's not what it should take.

To make matters worse, most student health departments don't have enough counselors to support the sheer population of students in need. A survey done by STAT news at Ithaca College found there were just two counselors to serve seven thousand students—an unsustainable student-counselor ratio (Thielking, 2017). Quality of services is another issue. Overworked and under-resourced counselors are unable to support students at the level they could if they had better training and lighter caseloads.

The mental health support staff at universities are seldom able to provide culturally competent care for increasingly diverse student bodies, growing year to year. Reduced budgets and overworked counselors make seeking consistent care nearly impossible. Therapy cannot be as effective without consistency, especially because developing a rapport with a therapist takes time. You need to consistently work with the same therapist for them to get to you and your background, as well as for you to get to know and be comfortable with them. Six sessions spanning the length of the academic year doesn't suffice. But for most students, it's their only option.

Mental health services on college campuses aren't really intended for long-term care either. They exist to help students deal with the ever-changing college environment. The issue is they are neither providing sufficient short-term care nor are they leaving a good impression on students. If an overtaxed college mental health system is someone's first exposure to therapy, they are unlikely to realize the substantial benefits that exist. Left with a bad taste in their mouth, they might be less willing to seek therapy post-graduation.

My own experience with therapy in college did little to convince me that therapy was worth pursuing post-grad. When I then attempted to do so in my early twenties, a complicated health insurance system stood as another barrier. That's not a problem specific to South Asians, though. The resource guide in the Appendix has more on this.

The issues I have highlighted do not have simple fixes. These require substantive investment in mental health services across the board. There are things we can do, however, to mitigate these hurdles and make therapy work for us. At the end of the day, therapy is a service you seek and, just like any service, you should do your homework to find the version that is the best fit for you. "Try out" your therapist and if you don't feel comfortable with them, move on. While it's not ideal to have to reintroduce yourself to another practitioner, you will save yourself from wasted time and money on a provider who isn't working for you.

When shopping around for therapists, schedule an initial consultation call to get a better understanding of their approach and style. Use this conversation to describe what you are looking for and determine whether that fits with their methodology and areas of expertise. If cultural competency is as important to you as it is to me, bring this up. During my initial conversation with a therapist, I brought up my previous negative experiences with therapists who lacked cultural competency. I explained how it was important for me that my provider understand while my culture and religion were a big part of my life, they didn't control every aspect of it. I needed my counselor to understand and be empathetic toward my cultural upbringing but not use it as a scapegoat for all my concerns. In my experience, I have found I am most comfortable with a therapist of color who doesn't share my cultural or religious background; you might find a shared background is necessary for you. I didn't go in knowing this, I learned by trial and error.

Find the environment where you feel the most comfortable sharing all parts of you. Remember the therapist can't help you with what they don't know is happening. If you aren't showing up authentically and honestly during therapy, chances are you won't see many of its benefits.

Therapy played a significant role in helping me take better care of my mental health. It even helped me conquer the imposter syndrome I felt when writing this book. It may not be something everyone is completely comfortable with at first. But the value of seeking therapy far outweighs the discomfort of being vulnerable.

Boundaries

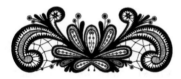

As we focus on protecting our mental health, a feeling of safety is requisite for us to process our traumas and begin healing. Setting boundaries is one way to create the safe emotional space necessary for the healing and rebuilding to occur. When I heard about the concept of setting boundaries, especially with family members, my first thought was: *This is only for white people whose parents allow these things; boundaries would never work in a brown family.* I was quite resistant to give the idea a second thought. Not only were boundaries such an alien concept, but they also seemed like a lot of hard work, and when you are already feeling unmotivated and depressed, hard work is the last thing you would want to do. I actually began to take pride in not having boundaries—*I don't need boundaries, I am an open book, there's no reason to hide things from people.*

The truth was I never completely understood what boundaries were and why being an "open book" (as I proclaimed to be) shouldn't absolve me from setting boundaries. In fact, boundaries aren't just about keeping personal information from others, nor are they meant to completely close you off from the world. Personal boundaries exist to help you flourish and feel secure in your relationships. Thoughtful, beneficial boundary-setting starts with understanding what boundaries really are and how exactly they are meant to help you.

WHAT ARE BOUNDARIES?

Boundaries are limits or rules *you* set for yourself within your relationships. "Boundaries are essentially about understanding and respecting our own needs, and being respectful and understanding of the needs of others," explains Stephanie Dowd, a clinical psychologist at the Child Mind Institute (Jacobsen, 2021). By setting boundaries, you're outlining what you're comfortable doing and what you're willing to accept from others. They work both ways—they protect you from other people and also other people from you. These "rules" allow you agency over your physical and emotional space. With this agency, you can be more comfortable in your relationships with others.

Generally, boundaries can be divided into a few categories:

- **Emotional:** These are related to feelings and emotions. You may also choose to set boundaries around how much you want to share your feelings or have others share theirs. This is usually a boundary you set for yourself.

For example, setting a limit on shouldering the burden of others' emotions.

- **Physical:** Including physical space as well as sexual boundaries, these have to do with your comfort level regarding your body. This can mean setting boundaries on what you are comfortable wearing, by whom or where you can be touched (hugging, kissing, etc.), or sexual acts you do or do not want to be involved in.
- **Time:** A boundary on your time can be set to delineate how much time you spend on various activities that are important to you. This can include work, religious activities, spending time with friends and family, hobbies, and self-care.
- **Material:** Material boundaries are related to your material possessions and how you would like others to interact with those things. This can also include your financial resources (setting a budget is setting a boundary on your financial resources).
- **Spiritual:** A spiritual boundary allows you to decide what role faith plays in your life and how you are comfortable interacting with it. Because religion, culture, and community are closely tied in South Asian households, setting spiritual boundaries can be especially challenging.

A key aspect about boundaries is they occur on a spectrum from loose to rigid. Kristina Virro, a psychotherapist, describes "when boundaries are loose, they're like lines in the sand and can change at any moment, and when they're rigid, they're like brick walls that do not budge" (Virro, 2020). You are not only able to decide which of your boundaries are loose or rigid, you can also decide when to change that. Different times of your life will require looser or more rigid boundaries, so you can (and should) adapt and change them as needed. "Healthy boundaries are firm yet flexible and keep our own feelings *and* other peoples' feelings in mind," says Varro. For example, during busy exam times in grad school, I changed my time boundaries to be more rigid. I reduced the amount of time I spent with friends or on leisure activities to accommodate my busier finals or midterm season. This proved to be difficult when the FOMO (fear of missing out) set in, but a big part of getting better at setting boundaries is to practice enforcing them.

BOUNDARIES FOR DESIS

Many Desis, like me, are resistant to setting or enforcing boundaries. It does not feel intuitive and sometimes feels plain wrong—especially when it seems like our boundaries might make others we love upset. Children learn social behaviors from their parents, and the truth is most of us have never seen boundaries in action. Our collectivist culture asks us to focus on others and their needs over our own. Witnessing our mothers wait to eat until after our fathers' bellies are full or our parents entertaining surprise guests late into the night on a work night taught us our own needs come second. You are praised and rewarded the more you can sacrifice your own self for others; it's a characteristic of good children, the *achay bachay* we were always striving to be. But this celebration of sacrifice and selflessness paves the way for us to become codependent in our relationships, feeling constantly compelled to please and serve others no matter the toll it takes on ourselves.

Growing up, I was a more adventurous eater than my siblings and would always want to try new restaurants. My picky sisters would never like any of the restaurants I wanted to go to and would get upset. Cue loud bickering and an upset dad. Dinner plans cancelled. My mom started taking me aside and telling me that as the big sister, it was my duty to sacrifice for the younger ones (*yeh badi behen ka farz hota hai*). I learned quickly. The next time my parents asked us where we wanted to go, I said I wanted to go Red Lobster, the only place they really liked. That time, and every time after, that was my answer and I was praised for it. By sacrificing my own needs for my sisters, I was a good sister. There was nothing wrong with me picking what they wanted sometimes, but doing so was *always expected* of me. Not once or twice, but **every** time. I learned then that I had to put my needs second. It mattered less what I wanted and more what others wanted.

Eating at Red Lobster didn't harm me, but it did negatively affect me when I began applying this principle to other parts of my life. Many of my boundaries (or lack thereof) were loosely set to easily accommodate the needs of others over myself. And being praised for forgoing my boundaries and needs when I was younger had me thinking I was doing the right thing. This is what I was taught, and was also what I saw my parents and cousins doing as well. As I now begin to set and enforce boundaries that prioritize myself, I'm slowly unlearning the mantras of self-sacrifice etched in my brain. Though, I still always have trouble picking a restaurant.

The process of setting boundaries is not intuitive for many South Asians. It did feel wrong to start doing so, and sometimes certain boundaries are still very uncomfortable for me to enforce. But learning a new skill takes time, as does unlearning harmful mindsets we were taught growing up. Just because it's difficult and uncomfortable now doesn't mean it will always be that way. Think back to the first time you drove a car. It was daunting, scary, and felt unnatural. *How am I maneuvering 1.5 tons of metal that could possibly kill me and others?* But you got better at it and more comfortable behind the wheel over time. All it really took was practice. Now being behind the wheel is as intuitive as walking. Boundary-setting is similar—it requires practice enforcing and setting boundaries to become better and more comfortable with them.

What scared me most about boundary-setting was having to enforce them, especially with my family. Enforcing boundaries meant having to reproach (potentially scold?!) others if they crossed a line, and that was a right I didn't think I had earned yet (at least not until parenthood). *Would I have to shut out everyone who didn't understand or respect my boundaries? Would I even have anyone left after that?*

Much of the western narrative surrounding boundaries (especially on social media) advises us to cut people off if boundaries are crossed. Not only is this extremely difficult to do in a collectivist culture, but it wasn't something I—or us Desis—want to do. So I had decided it was more important to maintain my family relationships than to set boundaries with my family. That is where I was wrong. It is entirely possible to set and enforce personal boundaries in a Desi family. For us, it will require a lot more communication and a slower journey. The approach will look different from what your non-Desi peers may have experienced, especially because this concept is new to us. Start this conversation by first addressing why setting boundaries are important to you and your mental health.

WHY ARE BOUNDARIES IMPORTANT?

One misconception I held onto for a long time was that setting boundaries was selfish. Growing up in our collectivist culture, saying "no" to family members or not wanting to discuss certain things was not permissible. The few times I used the phrase, "I don't want to talk about it," I was reprimanded for not sharing my concerns because "That's not how it works with family." Many of us were denied the opportunity to build or even understand what boundaries were. They were made out to be a selfish act. But the truth is, creating and enforcing boundaries ***does not*** make you selfish! It is not selfish to establish limits for yourself and how you want to be treated. Boundary-setting is a form of respecting and honoring yourself (and others).

Boundaries help make you have what you need to be comfortable in your relationships with others. In an airplane, we're always told to, in case of an emergency, put our oxygen masks on first before helping others. You cannot show up fully and comfortably for those around you without making sure you have what you need first, *your* oxygen mask. Think of boundaries in the same way. By not setting boundaries, we essentially ignore our own needs for others. Take it from someone who has spent most of her life doing that—it's not sustainable and actually hurts your relationships. Setting and enforcing boundaries is an act of self-care and self-protection, not an act of selfishness. Author of *Setting Boundaries*, Dr.

Rebecca Ray reminds us that boundaries empower us and help us prioritize what is important. By setting and enforcing them, you are demonstrating to others how they can respect you and how you respect yourself—your time, your body, your emotions, and your energy.

Typically, boundaries have to do with how you interact with others or how they interact with you. But to truly practice self-care (which boundaries are a part of), it's equally important to set boundaries with your own self. As a child, many of us longed for the freedom we thought adulthood would bring—a chimera. When we went away to college, we tried to take advantage of the new independence we had, no longer being ruled by the phrase, "You can do that after you get married." Many of us did not know how to act with the limitless sovereignty we suddenly had. Several of my peers described "going crazy" during college in hopes to make up for lost time from the restrictions of immigrant households. Because South Asian children tend to grow up in overly strict settings, we took our freedom to the extreme and decided boundaries (of any sort) were unnecessary. We disregarded our physical and emotional health, desperate to soak up everything freedom had to offer. It wasn't healthy. What we lacked were boundaries with ourselves, something we were unaware we actually needed until we didn't have any.

Taking care of yourself also requires setting limits for yourself. This keeps us safe and healthy, our lives running smoothly. For example, you can set boundaries with yourself on how much TV you watch or social media you consume. You can set a boundary on how many nights a week you go out, spend money, drink alcohol, or whichever other limits you think would help you be healthier. Boundaries are self-care. They give you the agency in your life to make the best choices for yourself. Isn't that the independence we always wanted growing up?

Jessie Dhaliwal, a trauma-informed counselor, described to me the importance of creating boundaries in the healing process as well: "Boundaries help you create space to preserve your energy while you are going through the trauma-healing process." Healing from trauma requires a level of safety and comfort in your surroundings: a space where your experience is not denied so you can grieve what you have lost. "The healing process is not just about what the trauma physically took from you, but the other experiences it also robbed you of while you were experiencing and coming to terms with it," Dhaliwal said. With the space you gain from setting boundaries, you are able to grow and improve your mental health. By creating boundaries, we are essentially giving ourselves the space to deal with the mental health concerns we have so we can move forward and reconnect with others.

HOW TO SET BOUNDARIES?

Whether we have explicitly stated them or not, we all have boundaries. There are things we're comfortable doing and things we aren't. Where it often gets tricky is enforcing and communicating boundaries, especially with loved ones. The boundary-setting process is about being more intentional with the boundaries you do have and evaluating your life and relationships to see if there are other boundaries you may need. The following steps can help you be more intentional about setting, enforcing, and communicating your limits with others.

IDENTIFY THEM

As you embark on the boundary-setting journey, start by identifying your needs and comforts. Think about your relationships (you, friends, family, partners, coworkers) and how you feel when interacting with others. Are there moments or interactions that make you uncomfortable?

Ask yourself some of these questions and write down the answers. I have always found writing down my thoughts and answers to even the most complicated questions helps me process them better:

- What are my rights?
- How do I want to be treated by others?
- What are things I am not comfortable with doing (or saying) or other people doing (or saying) to me?
- What are some boundaries I already have? Are they healthy? Unhealthy?
- When have people violated a boundary? What did I do about it?
- What are some healthy boundaries I can set for myself?

With the answers to these questions, you'll get a better idea of the boundaries you have and may need to set.

COMMUNICATE AND ENFORCE THEM

If you want others to respect and follow your boundaries, you must communicate that to them. This is a key step in the process. Verbally and explicitly communicating your boundary to others about what you expect from them will prevent misinterpretations of your limits. Therapist Nedra Tawwab provides an example of verbally communicating your boundaries: "'It's important to me that you honor plans we set up. If you need to change our plans, please send me a text a few hours before'" (Tawwab, 2021). By explicitly mentioning the behavior you are not okay with, you let the other person know how they can change their behavior to better suit your needs.

When communicating your boundaries, it's important to be explicit and assertive. Use "I" statements that help identify what you *feel* and what you *need*:

> "I feel_____when_____because_____.
> What I need is_____."

Asserting your needs can be difficult with South Asian families. When communicating your boundaries with your family, you may have to use different language or approaches to factor in cultural norms. Use the language and approach you know will work best for your family. For example, some parents are more partial to statistics, others are more convinced by personal anecdotes. It isn't a one-size-fits-all approach. It's a process and it takes time.

Start by easing your family into the idea of setting boundaries. This is probably a completely foreign concept to them, and you should expect some discomfort in the beginning. By communicating smaller boundaries or requests first, you can help your family understand the necessity and importance of setting boundaries. As they become more comfortable with you communicating your limits and needs, you can address boundaries that might be more inflexible or controversial to discuss. Our parents and families are usually willing to give us what we need as long as they understand where those needs are coming from. Being gentle and open about your needs will help everyone see you are ultimately trying to protect yourself and your relationships.

If someone has violated a boundary you have communicated to them, you should take action and address it. You need to let the other person know 1) a boundary was violated, 2) how it affects your relationship, and 3) how you can move forward and amend the situation. Try to do this when the situation occurs so you can be sure it doesn't repeat itself, that you don't hold resentment toward this person before having the discussion, and so they're better able to remember the incident. By enforcing your boundaries with other people, you are holding yourself, as well as others, accountable to the boundaries you have set. You are stating you take your boundaries seriously and it matters to you how others respond to those boundaries. This will help you ensure others are respecting your limits and make your relationships stronger. On the other hand, if someone has been doing a great job of respecting your boundaries, express your appreciation. This will also show it does matter to you that your boundaries are respected.

Due to the COVID-19 pandemic, I spent half of my last year of grad school living at home with my parents. I would spend my days in classes, doing assignments, and having meetings for projects (and writing this book) in my room. Every so often I would come upstairs to grab a snack, walk around a bit, or just to take a brain break. When my dad would see me upstairs, he would ask me to help out with an e-mail or try to strike up a conversation. I started to respond apathetically or would quickly find an excuse to go back to my room. My dad would get upset that I was being rude and ignoring him. I then stopped taking my break because it seemed to end in me being frustrated rather than relaxed. I realized I had not set a boundary with my dad about my work schedule. He did not know when I came upstairs for a few minutes, that was my break time and not a signal I was free for the day. I sat him down and communicated my boundary with him:

"Dad, whenever I need a break in my workday or just want to walk around for a bit, I come upstairs for a little bit. I usually limit this break time to ten or fifteen minutes because I know I still need to get back to my work and meetings. I appreciate our conversations and want to chat with you during that time, but I also want to make sure I don't stay longer than the break time I allotted for myself. If there's something you need from me, I'd be happy to help you when I'm done with my work for the day. I can come upstairs and tell you when I've signed off and don't have any more meetings or work to finish that day."

After this conversation, my dad was more mindful of my break times and I was more at ease when chatting with him during my breaks. He would even remind me when my time was up, helping me stay accountable to the boundary I had set for myself.

While this conversation was not too difficult after I explained my feelings, other boundary conversations might be more difficult. Approaching our parents from a place of grace and patience will also limit misinterpretations when discussing boundaries. Change is hard for everyone. The lack of boundaries we grew up with is a cultural phenomenon passed down through the generations. It isn't easy to unlearn these inherited behaviors—but it's not impossible.

REEVALUATE THEM

As I mentioned before, most boundaries are not steadfast (though some, like certain physical and sexual boundaries, can and should be). They change over time, just as your needs do. As you go through the healing process and deal with your anxiety, depression, or other mental health issues, you may decide specific boundaries you had set are no longer necessary. Or you may decide you need to add a new boundary based on a new situation. You can shift and change your boundaries as you go, so long as you communicate those changes to those around you.

Remember the boundary-setting journey is not going to happen overnight. Dr. Rebecca Ray aptly states: "Boundaries trigger complex feelings within us and sometimes, challenging responses in others" (Ray, 2021). Learning something new is never instantaneous, especially when it clashes with or challenges your previous beliefs and habits. As you practice setting boundaries, you will get better at doing so over time. It will become more natural and comfortable each time you do it. Every time you are successful at setting and enforcing a boundary, acknowledge that growth and milestone. Your journey to take care of yourself and protect your mental health is always worth celebrating!

Difficult Conversations

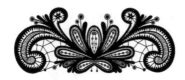

When I first spoke up about mental health with my family and even friends, I simultaneously felt relieved and terrified. I felt a weight off my shoulders, but still had a lump in my throat. It was relieving to name and identify what I was feeling out loud. I would no longer *need* to make excuses. But now I no longer *could* make excuses—there was no taking back what I said. While it was an uncomfortable and daunting conversation to have, it was also a necessary one. Talking about my mental health allowed me to come to better terms with it for myself. I was even able to help my family learn about and understand this foreign concept in their own way and in their own time. After several conversations over many years, they've grown to be better informed about mental health and how to take care of it. At the very least, they believe it exists and know it can't just be prayed away.

The only way to truly break the stigma and normalize conversations about mental health is to talk about it, especially with our parents and communities. It's difficult and it's uncomfortable and it will be the last thing you want to do, especially when you may already be dealing with poor mental health. But the alternative is much worse. Having this conversation is not just about bringing awareness to this topic. This is about creating space for others to feel less alone as they struggle with an experience that already leaves them despondent. This conversation can open doors to find new ways to take care of ourselves and each other. If we never have this conversation, we may not realize others are hiding the same struggles we are behind the "I'm fine's" and "I'm okay's."

BUILDING BLOCKS OF DIFFICULT CONVERSATIONS

Difficult conversations happen every day: between colleagues at work, spouses at home, and friends at school. They're the conversations we enjoy the least and put off the most. They cause anxiety and may strain our relationships—of course they're not fun. Enjoyable or not, difficult conversations are necessary for us to have, especially when it comes to talking about mental health with our South Asian families.

In their book *Difficult Conversations*, Douglas Stone, Bruce Patton, and Sheila Heen provide a roadmap to discuss what matters most. Their model for having difficult conversations is a useful tool to better understand and approach a challenging conversation. They start by revealing every difficult conversation is actually three conversations:

- **The "What Happened?" Conversation:** The difficulty here is nailing what happened, what should have happened, and who is to blame.
- **The Feelings Conversation:** Set in the background, each participant brings their emotions about the situation into the conversation.
- **The Identity Conversation:** This is an internal conversation each participant has with themselves about their identity and what the situation may reflect or change about their identity.

Within these three parallel conversations, we tend to make many assumptions and misjudgments that end up making our conversations more difficult than they have to be. In the "What Happened" Conversation, people often differ in their interpretation of the facts at hand and what is important. Interpretation is rooted in identity so it's necessary to consider the other party's view of the situation as well as your own. Our families' interpretation of our struggle with mental health and its roots comes from a very different perspective than our own. "What happened" according to them is very different from what we believe happened. When both parties fail to acknowledge that, it is hard to productively move the conversation forward.

Conversation can also become challenging when people assume the worst about others' intentions. We base these suspicions on our own feelings and jump to the assumption they have bad or hurtful intentions. Our understanding of the other party's objectives heavily influences our judgment of them and the situation. Stone and his colleagues state, "We make an attribution about another person's intentions based on the impact of their actions on us. We feel hurt; therefore, they intended to hurt us" (2003).

When we assume the worst on behalf of the other party, we end up leaping to the conclusion that they have bad character. We get defensive. They get defensive. We end up talking over each other, no one really hearing what anyone is really trying to say. We tend to project our own anxieties, fears, and biases as assumptions on the other person. When we're assuming something about someone, it's usually more about us than them. So, when our parents make assumptions about us, that's often coming more from their fears and anxieties about what could happen than what they actually believe did happen. When having the mental health conversation with our parents, it's especially important to disentangle their intent from their impact. Start by forming a hypothesis (a guess) about their intentions based on: 1) what they said or did, 2) how it impacted you, and 3) what you are assuming their intention to be. It is then imperative to share this hypothesis with them and inquire about their intentions. Don't assume.

In talking about what happened, blame is always central to the conversation. *Difficult Conversations* remind us "focusing on blame is a bad idea because it inhibits our ability to learn what's really causing the problem and to do anything meaningful to correct it" (2003). Blame immediately puts everyone on the defensive and breaks down meaningful communication. It's very easy, in our case, to blame our parents, our cultures, or our religions as the cause for all our problems. The solution here is to focus on outlining each party's *contribution* to the situation. By acknowledging the various contributors to a situation, we can proactively find solutions to the issue at hand. When the contribution of blame is divided among several parties (people or otherwise), it's easier for all parties to accept their contribution rather than the entirety of the blame. This puts everyone involved at ease and less likely to become defensive.

The Feelings Conversation is an inevitable part of any difficult conversation. Both expressed and concealed emotions are always at work in our interactions, and it is necessary to acknowledge them. Especially in the case of mental health, feelings are often what cause more friction than the actual issue itself. First, we must understand our own feelings as they relate to the situation. This requires a bit of self-reflection and, more importantly, honesty. If you are feeling hurt, upset, or offended by something, admit that to yourself! These feelings are usually hiding in plain sight and will eventually find their way into the conversation, invited or not. It is best, then, to give these feelings a voice and talk through them. If not, unspoken feelings will show up in our body language, tone, and facial expression. Also, "unexpressed feelings can block the ability to listen," preventing any productive conversation (Stone et al, 2003). As you reflect on our feelings, think about a few things:

- What specifically am I feeling? *Use a* Feelings Wheel *(see Appendix) to decipher whether your anger, for example, is really coming from feeling frustrated or disrespected.*
- How are these feelings affecting my judgment about this other person and their role in this situation?
- Did this situation intensify or reveal something I was already feeling?

- If this is how I am feeling, how might the other party be feeling?

These questions can help you take stock of your feelings while also considering the feelings of the other person. If you're feeling something, so are they. You might even find the root of the problem hidden beneath the surface of accusations and blame.

Perhaps the most important and consequential of the three conversations, the Identity Conversation, is the reason we must have the difficult conversation in the first place. Stone and his colleagues aptly remind us that "before, during, and after the difficult conversation, the Identity Conversation is about what I am saying to myself *about me*" (p. 14). When speaking with your family and loved ones about mental health, the Identity Conversation will be the most salient. These conversations are difficult specifically because our identities are reflected in them and their outcome. If we are talking about struggling with our mental health or discussing seeking therapy, our identities are bound to be at the center of the conversation.

PATHWAYS THROUGH A DIFFICULT CONVERSATION

Keeping the principles of *Difficult Conversations* in mind, I present a pathway on how we can break the stigma and have the mental health conversation with our South Asian families. A recurring theme during my interviews was how powerful these conversations can be, how they can really move the needle. We've been afraid of talking about mental health for so long, we have rehearsed this conversation and thought about the hundreds of (scary) possibilities. But we might be overestimating the size of the monster under this bed. Below I have outlined five steps to have this difficult conversation with our family and loved ones:

1. SELF-REFLECTION:

Start with deciphering where you are in the process and what you need from this conversation. Think about your journey with mental health so far: What has it been like? Have you had others to lean on? What have you learned throughout the process? When discussing your mental health with your family, you will likely be asked similar questions about your journey. You'll be more prepared to answer those questions after having thought, or journaled, about it first.

Some of these questions might even bring up triggering memories since you're being asked to relive your difficulties with mental health. This might be a time to work with a therapist on coming to terms with and better understanding yourself. When self-reflecting, consider your boundaries and what you're comfortable discussing (and what you're not).

One of my own anxieties when having this conversation was I wouldn't be able to take it back once it was out there. Make sure you understand the risks involved with having this conversation. The outcome of your discussion could likely change your family dynamic. If you can, discuss those risks and potential strategies to cope with a therapist or trusted confidant.

Next, think about what your goals are for this conversation. Are you simply looking to share something or are you looking for a specific type of support? Both of those conversations would go quite differently, so it's important to have a clear goal in mind. If it helps, write out a list of what you hope to achieve through the conversation as well as from the various family members you are talking to.

2. COME PREPARED:

You must do your homework and you must do it thoroughly. This is not something you can or should half-ass. The more prepared you are for this conversation, the better the outcome will potentially be. Preparation will help reduce the anxiety you might be having about the conversation: you will feel more confident if you're prepared with the answers to their questions.

Your biggest advantage going into this conversation is the sheer amount of information you already have available about your family. You've known your parents and family your entire life. You know what they like and dislike. You know how they process information. You know their background, their story, their triggers. Use this information to your advantage! If your parents like numbers and data, bring numbers and data. If they're more inclined to understand by example, find examples that support your case. If they're more religiously inclined, bring that into the conversation to help support you. Most importantly, you know best what your parents will find disrespectful and when they might shut down (the Feelings Conversation). Do your best to avoid those triggers for a more productive conversation.

Bringing up topics that your parents are both unfamiliar and uncomfortable with necessitates data and evidence to back up your stance. Do your research on the symptoms you're experiencing and what they mean. Many mental health advocacy organizations have parent-facing literature and informational materials (some of these are even available in different languages). Most Desi families are inclined to believe in science and doctors, bringing in statistics from medical professionals will likely help your argument. Bringing in facts, statistics, and research will help you back your claims and give your parents a perspective they may not have considered. The more you approach this conversation from a factual standpoint, the more effective you'll be.

Go one step further than researching facts and statistics. Depending on what your goals are for the conversation, do some legwork in advance. If you're looking to incorporate a new self-care practice that you might need permission for, bring specific plans. If you're looking to seek therapy, bring information on specific therapists or even schedule an informational interview with a therapist. Bring reviews of the therapist, what they specialize in, and their credentials. Having this information already available shows you not only thought long and hard about this, but you're confident and sure in describing your needs.

Simply having a conversation around mental health for awareness will definitely help to shift your family's mindset. But if you're specifically struggling with your mental health, the conversation might focus more on what you need to take care of yourself. In that case, you'll want to make sure you come to the conversation prepared with a solution or two. Think about what exactly you need from your parents. Is it support or permission to seek therapy? Is it space to practice self-care? Are you trying to set boundaries that you need them to understand? Desi parents are typically more action-oriented, so you'll want to make sure you discuss what you need from them moving forward.

3. MAP OUT THE LOGISTICS:

Logistics are often overlooked, but they can sometimes make or break a conversation. The location, time, and atmosphere can either make the conversation more difficult or help it be more productive. Think about these logistics in advance and use them to your advantage.

When finding a time, make sure no one will be in a rush or distracted due to other obligations. You want those involved to give you their full, undivided attention. Find a place where everyone can feel comfortable and stay focused on the conversation. While it may feel easier, bringing up this important conversation while family members are cooking or cleaning won't create the atmosphere you need. Sit your family down with intent: you need this time to discuss something important. Find a time and space where interruptions will be minimal, keeping the focus on the conversation.

You may want to have this conversation with certain family members at different times or without others present. Plan it out so only those you want to have this conversation with are in the room. You don't want to feel rushed or be nervously looking over your shoulder for unwanted participants. It's also best to find a time when folks aren't hungry, stressed, or tired. When our physical needs are not met, we tend to be less rational and may get upset faster than usual (you definitely don't want anyone to be hangry).

Any time you are going into a tough conversation, I recommend preparing an exit strategy beforehand. This discussion will be difficult and emotionally taxing. Based on the boundaries you have set up for yourself, you'll know if you're reaching your limit and when continuing the conversation will become too laborious. An exit strategy is something that will help you end the conversation and physically leave the situation. This can be a statement that helps proactively cut the conversation short if you think it's not productive:

> *I think we would both (all) benefit from taking a break to think about what was said today. We should continue this conversation another time, after we have had time to process.*

4. USE YOUR SUPPORT NETWORK:
Use your therapist, friends, teachers, and other mentors in your network as confidants. Practice your conversation or go over the points you plan to cover with someone. This will give you another perspective on your conversation and how it might be interpreted. Your network might be able to give you some feedback and help you anticipate questions that might get asked. Think of it like a presentation you have to give for class or work and consider it a dry run. By practicing with your support system, you'll feel more confident and better prepared going into the actual conversation.

You can also lean on this network if your conversation doesn't go as planned. Knowing you're having this conversation with your family, your therapist or friends can be there afterward to help you talk through how the conversation went and what you can do to move forward from it.

5. PACE YOURSELF:

The conversation surrounding mental health will not happen in one sitting, nor should it. This is a recurring conversation, a learning conversation that takes time. Your family and parents may not understand it fully the first time, but if they're willing and seeking to understand your perspective, that is already a great start. Remember they aren't familiar nor comfortable with discussing issues of mental health. It will take time and more exposure to bring a more permanent mindset shift.

There's also a chance this conversation doesn't go the way you want it to. You might experience pushback and find people unwilling to step out of their comfort zone to listen. In that case, you want to make sure you do what you can to protect your mental health and know when it's time to step back. During this process, you will need to be attentive to your self-care needs (as having this conversation may trigger past trauma or be traumatic itself). If you feel like you won't be able to make progress and get through to them, there is nothing wrong with ending the conversation.

What is still necessary is you working to protect your mental health—with or without the support of your family. Their support, while ideal and helpful, isn't necessary for you to do what is best for you. If that is the situation you find yourself in, work on setting boundaries with them. Think about how you can maintain a relationship while still prioritizing your mental health. That relationship might not look the way you anticipated, but by setting your boundaries, you will be doing your mental health a favor. And that is something you deserve.

The Charge Ahead

Dear Future Generation,

Today, we write to you the letter we wish our parents had written us. Our parents, from the sandwich generation, didn't know better. They weren't raised to be the parents we needed. Afraid, alone, and lost, they did the best they knew to do.

But we know better—better because we learned, firsthand, the power a parent's words hold. We witnessed the consequences of passing down a culture rooted in trauma.

We can be and do better, for you. We won't be perfect, but we promise to do right by you.

We made it through the criticisms, the guilt-tripping, the emotional blackmail. We survived the *Log Kya Kahenge* apocalypse. We came out the other side and stood up against the toxic masculinity and patriarchal gender norms. We, the poster children, did whatever we could to live as authentically as possible. We had the difficult conversations with our families, and we set our boundaries. We practiced self-care to protect our mental health. Some of us even went to therapy.

And we did it all for you. Because now, we know better. And now we can teach you how to be better too.

Love,
Your Brown Mothers (and Fathers)

P.S. We promise to love you exactly as you are, unconditionally and without judgment.

Your ceiling is the next generation's floor.

-ERIC THOMAS

Through the letters and the narrative I shared with you, I'm hoping the necessity of discussing mental health in the South Asian diaspora communities is glaringly obvious. Addressing this with our families and communities is the first step to collectively heal from the generational trauma and toxic facets of our culture. It's only by talking about this can we destigmatize mental health and normalize seeking help when it is needed.

All of our families will be in different places on this journey, but it is a journey we must take together as a collective South Asian community. It's not too late to remove the stigma on mental health yet. But, soon it will be. If the pandemic has shown us anything it's that mental health cannot be ignored any longer.

This isn't only for us—this is for the next generation of kids *we* will bring into the world. It's up to us to create spaces for them to feel loved, welcomed, appreciated, and heard. Just as our parents wanted for us, they deserve the best. And with the resources, knowledge, and experiences we've accumulated, we're equipped to give them that.

Generations of cultural practices and systems can never be uprooted overnight. But they *can* be changed. They *can* evolve for the better. As I've been discussing this topic with others over the past year, I've already seen the tide starting to shift. We're starting to stand up for ourselves and our mental health. The road ahead is long, and it'll be tough for many of us. **This is when resilience is crucial.**

Despite the trauma and stigma, we do have what it takes to conquer this challenge. I've seen this resilience in every story I heard throughout this process. Each of them found a way to move forward and reconcile their mental health. They may not have started in the same place or dealt with the same things, but they each left me with a message and feeling of hope: hope that we would be the last ones to suffer in silence; hope that the next time someone struggled with their mental health, they wouldn't have to fight alone; and hope that this stigma would be gone once and for all. This time *we* get to write the rules, and I hope we can do better for ourselves and for our future generations.

Glossary

abu ab-boo | father • other variations include: papa, baba, bapu, baap, aba, pita-ji, peo

achay bachay u-chay bu-chay | good kids • in order to be this you had to do as you were told and never step a toe out of line • you could either be this or be who you are, there often isn't room for both • this is overrated

anxiety | a mental health disorder characterized by feelings of worry, anxiety, or fear that are strong enough to interfere with one's daily activities • can be paralyzing • there's always something to worry about

ammi uhm-me | mother • other variations include: ma, mama, amma, mata, bebe, mummy

aunties | used to collectively refer to the women our mothers' age in the community • our mom's friends • our mom's competition • they always have some gossip

apne budhe baap ko nahi bhoolna up-nay bhud-dhay baap ko nu-he bhool-na | don't forget about your aging father • what they really meant was: you owe your parents your life, you'll never be able to repay them for that; don't forget

bechara(m)/bechari(f) bay-cha-ra/bay-cha-ree | poor thing, pity • if you're a girl, they'll always pity you for not being married

balla buhl-la | bat used to play cricket • sometimes used in case of misbehavior by children

beta bay-tah | son • also used as a gender-neutral term to address your child

beti bay-tee | daughter • seen as a liability if you have one

buzurk booz-ohrc | elders • many of them were wise and had great stories • some of them were too set in their ways and never accepted this new land as home

codependency | excessive emotional or psychological reliance on a partner, typically one who requires support on account of an illness or addiction

daal chawal thaal cha-vul | Rice and Lentils • poor man's food, because it's cheap and fills you up • the meal you always crave when you miss home • the first thing you learn how to cook

dada daaa-thuh | grandfather • other variations include: dadoo, dada abu, dada jaan, bade abu, nana, thakurda, darji

dadi daa-thee | grandma • other variations include: nani, dadi jaan, dado, bibi ji, baa, bebe, nanoo, daijan (dj)

desi they-see | people of South Asian descent • my people • representative of all our different countries, languages, cultures, religions, beliefs, and skin tones

depression | a mental health disorder characterized by persistently depressed mood, low self-esteem, loss of interest in activities, causing significant impairment in daily life • there are several types of depression • seasonal affective disorder (sad): experienced during winter months and triggered by seasonal changes • can be treated with medication

dramay-baaz dra-may baaz | dramatic • they think you're lying • they figured you're saying this for attention

enmeshment | description of a relationship between two or more people in which personal boundaries are permeable and unclear • over-concern for others leads to a loss of autonomous development

first generation | people born or raised in the united states, with at least one immigrant parent • this applies my sisters and myself • this also applies to my peers who may not have been born here, but were raised and grew up here

ghar ki izzat ka sawal hai ghur key ihz-zut ka sa-waal hai | it's a question of the family honor • isn't everything?

guriya goo-ree-ya | doll • what parents called their daughters lovingly sometimes

haan jee haan-jee | Yes, with reverence • if you didn't add the "jee" when speaking to your parents, you'd often get in trouble, especially when they were given you instructions for something

haandi haan-dee | any type of sauce-based dish or a clay pot, which curry is made in • there are more than one type of haandi • will make your house (and you) smell like curry powder, garlic, and onions • white kids will make fun of you for smelling like this at school • you'll hate eating haandi and want pasta for dinner instead; but Mom refuses to make that • when you grow up, you'll miss the taste and smell of mom's haandi

haath se nikal gaya(m)/gayi(f) haa-th say ni-kul ga-ya/ga-yee | he/she is getting out of hand or control • when kids start assimilating to American culture too much • parents assume this means you're on some road to destruction

immigrant generation | people born and largely raised outside of the United States to parents neither of whom was a US citizen, who immigrated to the US • this applies to my parents who immigrated from Pakistan

izzat ihz-zut | honor • rests on the daughter's shoulder • easily broken, never easily mended

jhootih(m)/jhootah(f) jhoo-teeh/jhoo-tah | liar • easy to call someone a liar when you don't want to believe them • this is how people gaslight you

joint-family system | an extended family arrangement consisting of many generations living in the same home, all bound by the common relationship • growing up with all your best friends (a.k.a. cousins) under one roof • the foundation of a toxic, controlling household environment where all members of your family (aunts, uncles, grandparents) dictate what you can and cannot do • the root cause of many marital and familial conflicts

kaafir kaah-fir | nonbelievers in Islam • you're immediately labeled this if you did anything deemed wrong or sinful

kismat kiss-muth | destiny • first thing to be blamed when things go badly • girls are considered to have bad kismat if they're not married by twenty-seven

kitty party kit-tee par-tee | a ladies-only social gathering • where Mom went to gossip and show off her childrens' accomplishments • where Mom brought home gossip from • where Mom started bringing rishtas for you • is this modern-day brunch?

lathi laa-teeh | a heavy stick often of bamboo bound with iron used as a weapon, especially by the police • used to control others

lgbtq+ | initialism used to refer to those who identify as lesbian, gay, bisexual, transgender, queer, intersex, or asexual • it's not a phase • you can't pray it away • you don't need fixing • love is love

log low-g | people, very nosy • everyone except whose business it actually is • they love to talk • they never look in their own backyards • it's usually the ones who you think would never spread any gossip

log kya kahenge lowg kyah ku-hai-n-gay | what will people say? • people always have something (negative) to say • this runs families more than the mard do • their conversations and accusations spread fast

mard mur-dh | man • the leader of the house • protector • there is no one way to be a man

mard ko dard nahi hota mur-dh ko dur-dh na-he ho-ta | men don't feel pain • but they do • doesn't make them any less manly if they do

mardangi mur-dan-gee | manhood • this seems to be threatened very easily

nakhre nukh-ray | being high-maintenance, being fussy, asking too much • if a girl shows nakhre, it's considered cute or flirty— sometimes • girls are expected to show some nakhre, other times they're shamed for doing so; they never tell you when the right time to show nakrhe is, but they expect you to know; it's usually always the wrong time

nazar nuh-zur | evil eye • also the first thing to be blamed when things go badly • jealous people will cast this on you if you're doing well in life • don't post anything good about yourself on social media, otherwise you'll get nazar • don't tell anyone, anything, ever • they're all out to get you

pagal pa-gull | crazy • attributed more frequently to girls and women • the easiest way to gaslight someone when they bring up a genuine mental health concern

patriarchy | a social system in which men (the father or eldest male) are head of the family and hold primary power and authority • Dad is king; he's always right • the root of a lot of the problems we face as a society • fuck the patriarchy

post-partum depression | a form of depression that occurs after childbirth • is not considered real in Desi families

post-traumatic stress disorder | a mental health problem that can occur after witnessing or experiencing a traumatic event including, but not limited to, war, assault, or disaster • symptoms can last months or years • triggers can bring back memories of the trauma • symptoms include nightmares, unwanted memories, avoidance of situations that might bring back memories, anxiety, or depression

roti row-tee | bread • your desirability as prospective wife or daughter-in-law is if your rotis are round • it takes a lot more practice than you think to make round rotis or even knead the dough properly • mom always uses her bare hands to flip them on the stove; you're always amazed and waiting until the day you can do that without being afraid

sabzi(s) sub-zee(s) | vegetables • you hated when Mom made those at home • usually looked down upon as a food category • Dad loved to eat these

second and higher generation | people born in the United States, with at least one parent born or largely raised in the United States • this will apply to mine and my sisters' future children

sharam shu-rum | modesty • girls are expected to have modesty in the way they dress, act, talk, breathe • used to shame you into submission

totka tote-ka | home remedies • usually involved putting some-thing smelly in your hair or eating something that tasted gross • they somehow always worked which was annoying because swallowing raw ginger and honey is not pleasant, but you'll do it anyways • I should write these down in a book or something

yeh badi behen ka farz hota hai yay ba-ri be-hen ka furz ho-tha hai | this is the duty of an older sister • these duties are almost the same as a mother's • it's a trap

Appendix

THE FEELINGS WHEEL

Our feelings may sometimes be difficult to recognize. They get jumbled together and can be elusive. Having a better and more targeted vocabulary to identify our feelings can help us better perceive the nuances with our emotions.

The inner ring is split into seven sections of emotions: Happy, Sad, Disgusted, Angry, Fearful, Bad, and Surprised. Though these specific emotions are easily identified and labeled, they are secondary to what you may actually be experiencing. The second and third rings of the wheel can help us find more accurate language for our emotions: I may identify feeling angry at first, but I might actually be <u>frustrated</u> or <u>annoyed</u>.

Use the Feelings Wheel here to effectively identify and artic-ulate your emotions.

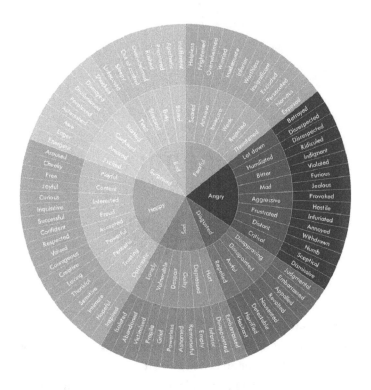

Originally created by Dr. Gloria Willcox (1982).

RESOURCE GUIDE

The *Letters to My Brown Mother* resource guide is filled with many different mental health resources for South Asian immigrants and children of immigrants.

To provide an easily accessible resource that can be regularly updated with new resources, I've created a digital guide available online.

Please check out the following link: https://linktr.ee/LTMBM

References

THE STIGMA

Center for Disease Control (CDC). "Leading Causes of Death Reports, 1981–2019." National Center for Injury Prevention and Control. Accessed August 22, 2020. https://webappa.cdc.gov/sasweb/ncipc/leadcause.html

Guha, Rohan. "Is It Time to Kill Off the Word 'Desi'?. *The Aerogram*. October 23, 2013. http://theaerogram.com/is-it-time-to-kill-off-the-word-desi/

Lamonier, Paulana. "My Black Is Beautiful - Reclaiming The Word And Redefining Beauty." *Forbes*. June 5, 2019. https://www.forbes.com/sites/plamonier/2019/06/05/my-black-is-beautiful-reclaiming-the-word-and-redefining-beauty/?sh=59a44304d901

Loya, Fred, Radhika Reddy, and Stephen P. Hinshaw. "Mental Illness Stigma as a Mediator of Differences in Caucasian and

South Asian College Students' Attitudes Toward Psychological Counseling." *Journal of Counseling Psychology* 57, no. 4 (2010): 484-490. doi:10.1037/a0021113.

Substance Abuse and Mental Health Services Administration. "Racial/ Ethnic Differences in Mental Health Service Use among Adults." HHS Publication No. SMA-15-4906. Rockville, MD: Substance Abuse and Mental Health Services Administration, 2015.

U.S. Department of Health and Human Services (US DHHS). "Mental Health: Culture, Race, and Ethnicity—A Supplement to Mental Health: A Report of the Surgeon General." Rockville, MD: U.S. Department of Health and Human Services, Substance Abuse and Mental Health Services Administration, Center for Mental Health Services, 2001.

ABCD | AMERICAN-BORN CONFUSED DESI

Das, Ajit K, and Sharon F Kemp. "Between Two Worlds: Counseling South Asian Americans." *Journal of Multicultural Counseling and Development,* 25, no. 1 (1997): 23–33. https://doi.org/10.1002/j.2161-1912.1997.tb00313.x.

Gorodnichenko, Yuriy and Gérard Roland. "Understanding the Individualism-Collectivism Cleavage and its Effects: Lessons from Cultural Psychology." In *Institutions and Comparative Economic Development,* edited by Aoki, Masahiko, Timur Kuran and Gérard Roland, 213-236. London: Palgrave Macmillan UK, 2012. doi:10.1057/9781137034014_12. https://doi.org/10.1057/9781137034014_12.

Heitzman, James, Robert L. Worden, and Library of Congress Federal Research Division. *India: A Country Study*. 5th ed. Vol. 550-21. Washington, D.C.: Federal Research Division, Library of Congress : For sale by the Supt. of Docs., U.S. G.P.O, 1996. http://hdl.loc.gov/loc.gdc/cntrystd.in; http://hdl.loc.gov/loc.gdc/scd0001.00205666473.

Ibrahim, Farah, Hifumi Ohnishi, and Daya Singh Sandhu. "Asian American Identity Development: A Culture Specific Model for South Asian Americans." *Journal of Multicultural Counseling and Development*, 25, no. 1 (January 1997): 34–50. https://doi.org/10.1002/j.2161-1912.1997.tb00314.x.

Kumar, Alok Prasanna. "The Right to Be Left Alone." *The Indian Express*, July 30, 2017. https://indianexpress.com/article/opinion/col-umns/aadhaar-card-data-privacy-the-right-to-be-left-alone-4774645/.

Maira Sunaina. *Desis in the House: Indian American Youth Culture in New York City*. Philadelphia: Temple University Press, 2002.

Mishra, Sangay K. *Desis Divided: the Political Lives of South Asian Americans*. University of Minnesota Press, 2016.

Nehru, Jawaharlal. *Toward freedom: The autobiography of Jawaharlal Nehru*. Boston: Beacon Press. 1963.

South Asian American Digital Archive (SAADA). "An Introduction to South Asian American History." Last Modified July 30, 2015. https://www.saada.org/resources/introduction

The Literary Digest. "Hindoos Too Brunette To Vote." *South Asian American Digital Archive.* https://www.saada.org/item/20101210-148. March 10, 1923.

THE INVISIBLE CRISIS

Das, Ajit K, and Sharon F Kemp. "Between Two Worlds: Counseling South Asian Americans." *Journal of Multicultural Counseling and Development,* 25, no. 1 (1997): 23–33. https://doi.org/10.1002/j.2161-1912.1997.tb00313.x.

National Alliance on Mental Illness (NAMI). "Mental Health By The Numbers." Last updated March 2021. https://www.nami.org/mhstats

Pew Research Center. *Second-Generation Americans: A Portrait of the Adult Children of Immigrants.* Washington DC: Pew Research Center, 2013.

Shannon-Karsik, Caroline. "Please Stop Thinking My High-Functioning Depression Makes Me Lazy." *Healthline.* Last reviewed June 20, 2017.

Soong, Jennifer and Michael Smith. "Depression Traps: Social Withdrawal, Rumination, and More." *WebMD* (April 2, 2014).

Weir, Kirsten. "The Roots of Mental Illness." *Monitor on Psychology,* 43, no. 6 (June 2012). https://www.apa.org/monitor/2012/06/roots

POSTER CHILD

Luyckx, Koen, Theo A. Klimstra, Bart Duriez, Stijn Van Petegem, Wim Beyers, Eveline Teppers, and Luc Goossens. "Personal Identity Processes and Self-Esteem: Temporal Sequences in High School and College Students." *Journal of Research in Personality* 47, no. 2 (2013): 159-170. doi:https://doi.org/10.1016/j.jrp.2012.10.005.

Samuel, Edith. "Acculturative Stress and Identity Crisis: South Asians in Canadian Academe." *Asian Journal of Social Science* 33, no. 2 (2005): 268-94. http://www.jstor.org/stable/23654362.

Shah, Sahil Ashwin. "South-Asian American and Asian-Indian Americans (SAA/AIA) Parents: Children's Education and Parental Participation." ProQuest Dissertations & Theses, 2015.

Shariff, Aneesa. "Ethnic Identity and Parenting Stress in South Asian Families: Implications for Culturally Sensitive Counselling." *Canadian Journal of Counselling* 43, no. 1 (Jan 1, 2009): 35.

LOG KYA KAHENGE | WHAT WILL PEOPLE SAY?

Chang, Hanna Yun-Han, "The Internalization of the Model Minority Stereotype, Acculturative Stress, and Ethnic Identity on Academic Stress, Academic Performance, and Mental Health Among Asian American College Students." Loyola University of Chicago Dissertations Publishing. 2017. https://ecommons.luc.edu/luc_diss/2785

Sathian, Sanjena. "How the Pressure of the Model Minority Myth Restricts Our Imagination—and Our Freedom." *Time.* April

9, 2021. https://time.com/5953333/model-minority-myth-re-stricts-inner-lives/

Smith, Disha. "Why I Was Disowned By My Family." *Disha Discovers* (blog). October 6, 2019. https://www.dishadiscovers.com/disha-discovers-being-disowned-by-her-family/

SANDWICH GENERATION

Ahluwalia, Jassa "Is enmeshment trauma a cultural norm in South Asian families?" *Burnt Roti* (Blog). May 13, 2020. https://www.burntroti.com/blog/is-enmeshment-trauma-a-cultural-norm-in-south-asian-families

Hooper, Lisa M., Sara Tomek, Justin M. Bond, and Meagan S. Reif. "Race/Ethnicity, Gender, Parentification, and Psychological Functioning: Comparisons Among a Nationwide University Sample." *The Family Journal* 23, no. 1 (January 2015): 33–48. https://doi.org/10.1177/1066480714547187.

LePera, Nicole. "Here's How To Tell The Difference Between Empathy & Codependency." *MindBodyGreen.* October 17. 2019. https://www.mindbodygreen.com/articles/difference-between-empathy-and-codependent-behavior-for-hsps

Love, Ryan. "Being the Eldest Child Is a Blessing and A Curse." *Independent.* August 7, 2014. https://www.independent.co.uk/life-style/health-and-families/features/being-eldest-child-blessing-and-curse-9651642.html

Preciado, Bertha, "Developmental Implications of Parentification: An Examination of Ethnic Variation and Loneliness." CSUB

Electronic Theses, Projects, and Dissertations. 1087. 2020. https://scholarworks.lib.csusb.edu/etd/1087

FAMILY HEIRLOOMS

Ahmed, Sumaiya. "Brown Girl Guilt." *Sumaiya Ahmed* (blog). March, 1, 2020. https://sumaiyaahmed.com/2020/03/01/ brown-girl guilt/?utm_medium=email&_hsmi=130966331&_ hsenc=p2ANqtz-87FfWZDGpJz7oJCNNKUR9NyShFgSb2I- Fey

Arnold, Fred, Sunita Kishor, and T. K. Roy. "Sex-Selective Abortions in India." *Population and Development Review* 28, no. 4 (2002): 759-85. Accessed July 2, 2021. http://www.jstor.org/ stable/3092788.

Brown, Brené. "Sham v. Guilt." *Brené Brown* (blog). January 14, 2013. https://brenebrown.com/blog/2013/01/14/shame-v-guilt

CBS. "Indian man accused of beheading teen daughter in apparent 'honor killing.'" *CBS News.* March 4, 2021. https://www. cbsnews.com/news/indian-man-accused-of-beheading-teen-daughter-in-apparent-honor-killing/

Christianson, Monica, Åsa Teiler, and Carola Eriksson. "'A Woman's Honor Tumbles Down on all of Us in the Family, but a Man's Honor is Only His': Young Women's Experiences of Patriarchal Chastity Norms." *International Journal of Qualitative Studies on Health and Well-being* 16, no. 1 (2021): 1862480. doi:10.1080/17482631.2020.1862480. https://doi.org/10.1080/174 82631.2020.1862480.

Kim, John M. "Asian Parents Who Say 'I Criticize Before I Care.'" *Asian Self-Help. Psychology Today.* May 27, 2020. https://www. psychologytoday.com/us/blog/asian-self-help/202005/asian-parents-who-say-i-criticize-because-i-care

Zaidi, Arshia U., Amanda Couture-Carron, and Eleanor Maticka-Tyndale. "'Should I Or should I Not'?: An Exploration of South Asian Youth's Resistance to Cultural Deviancy." *International Journal of Adolescence and Youth*, 21, no. 2 (2016): 232-251. doi:10.1080/02673843.2013.836978

MARDANGI | MANHOOD

American Psychological Association. "APA guidelines for psychological practice with boys and men." August 2018. https://www. apa.org/about/policy/boys-men-practice-guidelines.pdf.

Chakraborty, Souraja. "Mere pass toxic masculinity hain." *AlternateTake.* December 4, 2020. https://medium.com/alternate-take/-927d4cc74789

Desai, Mahmohan. *Mard.* 1985.

Gillette. "We Believe: The Best Men Can Be." January 13, 2019. Video. 1:48 https://www.youtube.com/watch?v=koPmuEy-P3ao&ab_channel=Gillette

National Eating Disorders Association. "Men & Eating Disorders." n.d https://www.nationaleatingdisorders.org/men-eating-disorders

Manzanares, Nina. "'Boys Will Be Boys' Gives Men a Pass on Accountability." *The Short Horn*, February 10, 2021. https://www.theshorthorn.com/opinion/opinion-boys-will-be-boys-gives-men-a-pass-on-accountability/article_bd877080-6b21-11eb-8130-83bc2f9f897c.html.

AMMI KI GURIYA | MY MOTHER'S DOLL

Kim, John M. "Asian Parents Who Say 'I Criticize Before I Care.'" *Asian Self-Help. Psychology Today.* May 27, 2020. https://www.psychologytoday.com/us/blog/asian-self-help/202005/asian-parents-who-say-i-criticize-because-i-care

Kohli, Sahaj (@SahajKohli). "This can also manifest as…" *Twitter.* December 9, 2020. https://twitter.com/SahajKohli/status/1336768135538544645

Indian Matchmaking. "Just Find Me Someone!" Netflix. Video. 33:32. 2020. https://www.netflix.com/title/80244565

Jayakumar, Nivedita. "Can A Toxic Mother Raise a Feminist Daughter?" *Feminism in India* (blog). February 14, 2020. https://feminisminindia.com/2020/02/14/toxic-mother-raise-feminist-daughter/

Martin, Sharon. "How to Break the Cycle of Codependency." *PsychCentral* (blog). September 22, 2017. https://psychcentral.com/blog/imperfect/2017/09/how-to-break-the-cycle-of-codependency

PRIDE

Alimahomed, Sabrina. "Thinking outside the rainbow: Women of color re-defining queer politics and identity." *Social Identities*, 16(2), (2010): 151–168. doi:10.1080/13504631003688849

Anwar, Kamillah (@Kamillahanwar), "Part One." *Instagram*. August 21, 2020. https://www.instagram.com/p/CELN-1HGhRwJ/

Bharat, Omsri. "Yoni Ki Baat: South Asian Queer Feminist Organizing." *Found SF* (blog). 2015. https://www.foundsf.org/index.php?title=Yoni_Ki_Baat:_South_Asian_Queer_and_Feminist_Organizing

Hinkson, Kasia. "The Colorblind Rainbow: Whiteness in the Gay Rights Movement." *Journal of Homosexuality* 68, no. 9, (2019): 1393-1416.

Patel, Sonali. "'Brown girls can't be gay': Racism experienced by queer South Asian women in the Toronto LGBTQ community." *Journal of Lesbian Studies*, 23, no. 3, (2019): 410–423.

Roberts, Andrea L, Margaret Rosario, Heather L. Corliss, Karestan C. Koenen, S. Bryn Austin. "Elevated Risk of Posttraumatic Stress in Sexual Minority Youths: Mediation by Childhood Abuse and Gender Nonconformity." *American Journal of Public Health* 102, no. 8 (August 1, 2012): pp. 1587-1593.

The Queer Muslim Project (@thequeermuslimproject). "Accepting myself as a…" *Instagram*. January 31, 2021. https://www.instagram.com/p/CKtZDO7FsaE/

SELF-CARE

Ali, Shainna. "Why Your Self-Care Isn't Working." *A Modern Mentality. Psychology Today.* January 6, 2019. https://browngirlmagazine.com/2018/09/self-care-is-not-a-luxury-how-i-learned-this-as-a-brown-guy/

Jacob, Steven. "Self-Care is Not A Luxury: How I Learned This As A Brown Guy." *Brown Girl Magazine.* September 2018. https://browngirlmagazine.com/2018/09/self-care-is-not-a-luxury-how-i-learned-this-as-a-brown-guy/

THERAPY

American Psychological Association (APA). "Protecting your privacy: understanding confidentiality." October 19, 2019. https://www.apa.org/topics/ethics/confidentiality

Hayes, Adele M., Jean-Philippe Laurenceau, Greg Feldman, Jennifer L. Strauss, and LeeAnn Cardaciotto. "Change is not always linear: the study of nonlinear and discontinuous patterns of change in psychotherapy." *Clinical psychology review,* 27(6), (2007): 715–723. https://doi.org/10.1016/j.cpr.2007.01.008

Jacob, Steven. "I'm a South Asian Guy in Therapy: Here's What Happened After 12 Sessions." *Brown Girl Magazine.* May 6, 2018. https://browngirlmagazine.com/2018/05/im-a-south-asian-guy-in-therapy-heres-what-happened-after-12-sessions/

Khan, Coco. "'I thought I was a lost cause': how therapy is failing people of colour." *The Guardian.* February 10, 2020. https://www.theguardian.com/lifeandstyle/2020/feb/10/therapy-failing-bme-patients-mental-health-counselling

Kim-Goh, Mikyong, Hyunmi Choi, and Myeong Sook Yoon. "Culturally Responsive Counseling for Asian Americans: Clinician Perspectives." *International Journal for the Advancement of Counselling* 37, no. 1 (2015): 63-76. doi:10.1007/s10447-014-9226-z.

Selva, Joaquin. "How to Become a Therapist." *Positive Psychology.* April 4, 2021. https://positivepsychology.com/how-to-become-a-therapist/

Sue, Derald and David Sue. *Counseling the Culturally Diverse: Theory and Practice*, 5th Ed. Hoboken, NJ, US: John Wiley & Sons, Inc, 2008.

Thielking, Megan "A Dangerous Wait: Colleges Can't Meet Soaring Student Needs for Mental Health Are." STAT News February 6, 2017. https://www.statnews.com/2017/02/06/mental-health-college-students/

Thomas, Julia, "Psychiatrist vs. Therapist: What's the Difference?" *BetterHelp* (blog). Updated June 24, 2021. https://www.betterhelp.com/advice/psychologists/psychiatrist-vs-therapist-whats-the-difference/

BOUNDARIES

Jacobsen, Rae. "Teaching Kids About Boundaries." *Child Mind Institute.* n.d. https://childmind.org/article/teaching-kids-boundaries-empathy/

Ray, Rebecca (@rrrebeccaray). "This goes for any…" *Instagram.* May 19, 2021. https://www.instagram.com/p/CPFGmYZsoH3/

Ray, Rebecca (@rrrebeccaray). "I've been doing some publicity…"
Instagram. May 25, 2021. https://www.instagram.com/p/CPU-naAOMRtt/

Tawwab, Nedra Glover. *Set Boundaries, Find Peace: A Guide to Reclaiming Yourself.* Penguin Publishing Group, 2021.

Virro, Kristina. "Boundaries 101." *Fresh Insight* (blog). August 17, 2020. https://www.fresh-insight.ca/post/boundaries-101

DIFFICULT CONVERSATIONS

Stone, Douglas, Bruce Patton, and Sheila Heen. *Difficult Conversations: How to Discuss What Matters Most.* New York: Penguin Books. 2003

Willcox, Gloria. "The Feeling Wheel: A Tool for Expanding Awareness of Emotions and Increasing Spontaneity and Intimacy." *Transactional Analysis Journal* 12, no. 4 (October 1982): 274–76. https://doi.org/10.1177/036215378201200411.

Acknowledgments

When I had the idea to write this book, I didn't realize I wouldn't be alone on this journey. *Letters to My Brown Mother* would not have been possible without the overwhelming love and support of my community. I'm so grateful for everyone who listened to my story and encouraged me to pour my heart into this book. Thank you for believing in me (even when I didn't believe in myself).

My dream to write a book is now a reality because of you all.

First, I'd like to thank my parents and family for everything I am today. Thank you for standing by my side and for your willingness to learn as I shared pieces of this book with you.

Thank you to my interviewees for sharing the personal stories and vulnerabilities that inspired the letters in this book. Your bravery and candor left me inspired.

Thank you to the readers for picking up and sticking with this book. I hope this book impacted in even the smallest of ways.

Thank you to my editor and my beta readers whose perspectives made this book stronger than I could have imagined: Ashley, Celia, Lavi, Vyasar, Saad, Fatima, and Youssef.

Thank you to Hafsa, HafandHaf, for bringing my vision to reality with your beautiful artwork on the cover of this book.

A special *no* thanks to my computer that made this process slightly more gruesome. Your loud engine-like roar did keep me company while I wrote and edited into the night, though.

Lastly, thank you to the supporters of my campaign who believed in my idea enough to finance it (in no particular order):

Nayab Abbas

Ghulam & Saniya Abbas

Kainat Abbas

Celia Laskowski

Paul J. Fischer

Lavanya Yeleswarapu

Mohamed Soltan

Teach For America Buffalo

Youssef Challita

Angela Park

Nirmal Patel

Aparna Sharan

Darshan Dholakia

Hiral Patel

Rizwan Lokhandwala

Julia Tvardovskaya

Shivani Patel

Amber Farid

Julia Tomaka

Joshua Caleb Parsons

Summer Kristine Quintana

Humaira Khawaja

Saurab Prabhakar

Mohammed Soliman

Anulekha Venkatram

Sahrish Baloch

Rubina Naureen

Vyasar Ganesan

Sonia Alam
Lauren Stephanie Hess
Priya Parikh
RJ Holmes-Leopold
Nicole Johnston
Judy Robinson
Stephanie Perera
Aminat Yahaya
Sadia Ilyas
Kimraj Jordan
Andrew Hart
Brian Wall
Katie Campos
Shanta Devarajan
Samantha Gressieg
Kevin William Russell
Saira Chaughtai
Taliha Yasin
Syeda Saba
Babar Baig
Iftikhar Khan and Family
Alina Shah
Sarah Van Horn
Aditi Soin
Maggie Chappel
Callie Marple
Claire A. Downs
Rohan Shamapant
Ryder Ashcraft
Shivani Parikh
Hamza Rubani
Jasmine Niazi

McLain Gore
Syed M. Razvi
Gabby Davidson
Nishaj Attassery
Rishad Mahasoom
Sheerin Vesin
Brendan Johnson
Eric Koester
Shahla Khan
Farzana Zaman
Jacky Contreras
Rabia Yasin
Henna Chaudhry
Shawn Mufti
Sofia Kaiser
Anishka Khosla
The Beg Family
Maitri Patel
Nighat Cheema
Anum Syed
Christiana Metaxas
Nicole Johnston
Luis M. Garzon-Negreiros
Bennie Williams
Obaid Syed
Hannah R. Richards
Lea Marich
Silvia Rodriguez
Alejandra Mendoza
Zaimah Khan
Nighat Bukhari
Cristine Starke

Mary Wall
Sidney Lynn
Karan Dholakia
Palak Mittal
Tierney Monahan
Austen Brower
Harini Sekar
Sravani Hotha
Priya Sirohi
Joann A. Harris
Braxton Bernard
Farheen Nabi
Coby Vail
The Rehman Family
Makala R. Forster
Nick Smith
Hozair M. Syed
Mohammad Amjad
Chaudhry
Tahira Shah
Menty Kebede
Elizabeth O'Neil
Amad Ali
Olga Thomas
Harris Masood
Ishanee Chanda
Elena Scott-Kakures
Hayley Rose
Scott Modesitt
Katie Quartuccio
Ilse Heine
Martina Senkyrikova

Faiza Susan
Abeera Jahangir
Kalif Robinson
Natasa Popovic
Saad Siddiqi
Salwa Saba
Chris Downs
Tim Kasckow
Alyssa Patricio
Shuaib Ahmad Shameem
Louie Limas
Sarah Wilcox
Kyoko Imai
Kumkum Mehta
Nick Weith
Rabia Yasin
Sana Siddiq
Mominah Farrukh
Raquel Villaba
Shahid Jamil
Karthikeya Easwar
Matt Johnson
Thamesha Tennakoon
Evelyn Nash
Divya Jethwani
Asma Qaiyumi
Mubaraka Mandviwala
Ashanka Kumari
Hareena Suprai

Printed in the USA
CPSIA information can be obtained
at www.ICGtesting.com
LVHW020245091123
763265LV00037B/1184/J